THE AGE-LONG HEALING SECRET WITH DMSO

KEISHA WRIGHT

All rights reserved. No part of this publication may be reproduced, distributed, or transmitted in any form or by any means, including photocopying, recording, or other electronic or mechanical methods, without the prior written permission of the publisher, except in the case of brief quotations embodied in critical reviews and certain other noncommercial uses permitted by copyright law.

Disclaimer:

The information contained in this book is for general informational purposes only. While every effort has been made to ensure that the content is accurate and up-to-date, the author and publisher make no representations or warranties of any kind, express or implied, about the completeness, accuracy, reliability, suitability, or availability of the information contained herein. Any reliance you place on such information is strictly at your own risk.

The content of this book is not intended to serve as professional advice or replace consultation with qualified professionals in relevant fields. The author and publisher disclaim any liability for any loss or damage arising from reliance on the information provided in this book.

INTRODUCTION 9

Understanding DMSO: The Science Made Simple 13

    What is DMSO? 13

    Why DMSO Remains a Hidden Gem 18

    How DMSO Works: Breaking Down the Science 22

    The Power of Penetration 24

Precautions and Considerations 27

    When and Why to Use Different Strengths? 27

    70-90% Concentration (The Powerhouse) 28

    50-70% Concentration (The Middle Ground). 29

    25-50% concentration (the gentle approach) 29

    Below 25% concentration (The Skin-Friendly Option) .. 30

    Potential side effects and how to avoid them. 31

    Skin irritation is the most common side effect. 31

    Garlic-Like Odor: A Quirky Side Effect 32

    Dry skin: A manageable issue. 32

    Safe Procedures for Internal and External Use 34

    External Use: Guidelines for Safe Application 34

    Internal Use: Proceed With Caution. 35

    General Safety Tips. 35

    Choosing the Right Grade of DMSO: What You Should Know 36

    Pharmaceutical-Grade DMSO in Healthcare 38

    The Versatility of DMSO: A Carrier of Health 39

    DMSO in Daily Life: Foods and Beyond 40

- Healing with DMSO: From Aches to Z 41
  - Arthritis Relief: Step-by-Step Guide 41
  - Skin Conditions: Eczema, Rashes, and More 44
  - Chronic Pain Management: Effective, Non-Addictive Solutions 46
  - Shield against the Invisible 47
  - Protecting Against Ionic Radiation 49
- Versatile Protector and Healer 51
  - How to Use DMSO Before and After Exposure 51
  - Before exposure 51
  - After Exposure 52
  - DMSO as a Lifelong Companion in a Toxic Environment 53
  - Works as an Anti-inflammatory Agent 55
  - DMSO: A Hidden Gem in Cancer Treatment 56
  - What Makes DMSO Stand Out? 57
  - DMSO's Effect on Leukemia Cells 58
- The Powerful Combo 59
  - DMSO and Cyclophosphamide 59
  - DMSO and the Immune System: An Important Ally 60
  - Hope for the Hopeless. 63
  - Why DMSO Should be an Important Part of Cancer Treatment 64
- Exploring DMSO for Diabetes Management 69
  - DMSO and diabetic neuropathy 69

Saving toes from amputation 70
Why DMSO Helps 71
The DMSO-Laetrile Combination 71
Unlocking the Potential of DMSO for Brain Health 79
Ear & Hearing Health: A New Approach 82
DMSO and Its Role in Arthritis 84
Boosting Recovery: How DMSO Can Transform Athletic Injury Treatment 89
Finding Relief: How DMSO Can Help with Digestive Troubles 94
Soothing Severe Burns: How DMSO Can Help 97
Finding New Hope for Liver Health with DMSO 99
Why DMSO should be a staple in emergency care 100
Managing Headaches with DMSO: A Unique Approach 103
Reviving Vision: How DMSO is Changing Eye Health . 105
Harnessing the Power of DMSO for Hair and Scalp Health 109
Fibromyalgia: A Personal Journey of Relief 111
Combating Fungus Infections: DMSO to the Rescue ... 113
Jungle Rot and its Remedies 113
Athlete's Foot and Foot Health 114
Treating Nail Fungus 114
Combating Foot Odor 115
Infections 116
Inflammation 117

Interstitial cystitis 120
The Power of DMSO Combinations 123
　DMSO in Black Salve... 124
　DMSO and Essential Oils 124
　Exploring essential oil combinations with DMSO 126
　Wintergreen Oil 126
　Peppermint Oil 127
　Black Pepper Oil 127
　Sweet Birch Oil 128
　DMSO and CBD Oil 128
　How to Use DMSO with Cannabis Extract 130
　Combining DMSO and Castor Oil 131
　How to Use DMSO with Castor Oil? 133
　DMSO with Colloidal Silver 134
　How to Use DMSO and Colloidal Silver 134
　DMSO with Botanical Medicine 135
　Using DMSO with Vitamin C: A Simple Guide 138
DMSO and MSM: A Powerful Healing Combination 143
　How to Use DMSO with MSM 144
　DMSO and Herbal Remedies: An Ideal Combination for Natural Healing 145
　Herbal Remedies: Nature's Medicine Cabinet 146
　Common Herbal Remedies: Combined with DMSO 147
　Safety Concerns and Precautions 149
　Acupuncture and DMSO: A Dynamic Duo. 149

Understanding Acupuncture 150
How DMSO Improves Acupuncture. 150
Combining Acupuncture with DMSO for Pain and Healing 151
Ayurveda and DMSO: Integrating Ancient Wisdom with Modern Science 152
What is Ayurveda? 152
Where Does DMSO Come In? 153
Practical Uses of Ayurveda with DMSO 154
DMSO and Physical Therapy: A Powerful Combination for Healing 155
What Physical Therapy Offers: 155
How to Integrate DMSO with Physical Therapy 157
A New Frontier in Natural Healing 159
How to Make and Use DMSO Eye and Ear Drops 163
Sinus Rinse 167
Wound Spray 168
Mouthwash 169
DIY Scalp Care and Hair Growth Spray 170
Topical Vitamin and Mineral Blend 172
Crafting Your Own DMSO Creams and Gels at Home 175
Choosing the Right Ingredients 175
Easy DIY DMSO Creams and Gels 176
Arnica-DMSO Cream: 177
Make Your DMSO Solutions at Home 178

Safety First: What You Should Know 180
Customizing Your DMSO Solutions 181
The Future of DMSO: Challenges and Opportunities. 183
Overcoming Legal and Medical Barriers 183
The Potential of DMSO in Modern Medicine 184
Advocacy and Education: How to Spread the Word ... 185
Conclusion 187

INTRODUCTION

Who would have thought that one of the most potent therapeutic medicines known to humans could be a basic compound taken from wood? Though it sounds implausible, you will probably agree after you learn about the science of DMSO (dimethyl sulfoxide) and hear the accounts of those who have had its amazing benefits. My journey with DMSO started with a great interest ignited during my employment in a natural health clinic, not with a particular illness.

One day, a patient arrived hobbling, her face contorted in agony. After hurting her knee on a hiking trip, she tried everything from over-the-counter medicines to ice packs but found nothing seemed to help. I recalled reading in a medical publication something about DMSO, a fleeting reference to its efficacy in reducing pain and inflammation. Intrigued, I advised her to try it. The result was virtually instantaneous: the swelling had gone down in minutes, and the discomfort had dropped sufficiently for her to stroll out of the clinic grinning.

This incident piqued my interest, but life continued, and so did I. DMSO disappeared from view as yet another cure, among others. Years later, having created many natural health products and extensively studied holistic medicine, I discovered I was at a crossroads. One evening, in sorting my workshop, I came upon an old DMSO bottle buried in a neglected corner. I felt a tsunami of recollections and decided it was time to investigate this material more closely.

Around that same period, a buddy of mine contacted me, clearly distressed. Her adolescent son suffered a serious allergic response, and hives covered his body. Though they had done everything, nothing appeared to make a difference. I hurried over right away with the DMSO. We applied it to the worst places, but we were unsure. The relief was clear-cut and quick. The hives started to fade, and within an hour, his skin was virtually normal once more.

For me, it marked a sea change. I realized that this wasn't just another remedy—DMSO was something extraordinary. I started researching nonstop, reading papers from decades ago, reading medical literature, and playing with different mixtures. What I found was really rather incredible. DMSO might stop heart attacks and stroke progression. It might ease suffering from dependency. It could even shield DNA from radiation without adverse effects.

I realized I had to impart what I had discovered. Combining my practical expertise in creating natural treatments with my knowledge in chemistry and holistic health helps me to grasp and communicate the miracles of DMSO. I began offering the world my expertise and excitement. The reply was really strong. People were keen to discover more and to know how this little liquid may have such great healing ability.

I grew more certain as I kept exploring and innovating with DMSO that this was a gift everyone should be able to access. Every family needs this item because it's a must-have in every first aid box. Surprisingly, even with its amazing advantages, DMSO is still mostly unappreciated and demonized in certain circles, especially in North America. I think that this comes from a mix of legislative limitations, false information, and ingrained medical practices opposed to reform.

This book is an effort at straightening the records. These sections include not just DMSO's background but also useful tips, recipes, and ideas on how you could use it for your well-being. This book will help you explore the various benefits of DMSO, whether your interests are in natural methods to improve your health, how to cope with chronic pain, or just discovering alternative medicine healing secrets. Let's travel this road together and find how a basic wood-derived compound could change life.

Understanding DMSO: The Science Made Simple

Dimethyl sulfoxide, or DMSO, has been regarded by its supporters (almost everyone who has ever tried it) as a real medical miracle. It has been utilized to cure hundreds of disorders that affect individuals across the world. In fact, DMSO, either alone or in combination with other drugs, has proven effective in the treatment of almost every known medical condition.

What is DMSO?

It is a natural chemical substance generated from trees as a byproduct of the paper-making process. It is made up of two methyl groups (CH3), a sulfur and an oxygen atom. In 1866, Russian scientist Alexander

Zaytsev synthesized it for the first time. For almost eighty years, DMSO was mostly overlooked. In the late 1940s, industrial chemists began researching the solvent properties of DMSO. Improved solvents were required, and there was interest in using tree-derived waste products.

Commercial development of DMSO began in the 1950s. Crown Zellerbach, a prominent American paper manufacturing corporation, began making DMSO about this period and eventually became the world's largest manufacturer. Robert J. Herschler was the supervisor of applications research at the Crown Zellerbach plant's chemical products section in Camas, Washington, just over the Columbia River from Oregon Health Sciences University. As a scientist, Mr. Herschler researched DMSO and other tree-derived compounds.

Stanley W. Jacob, M.D., was the chairman of the organ transplant team at the University of Oregon Medical School, now known as Oregon Health Sciences University. He wanted a mechanism to keep transplant organs at a low temperature without forming ice crystals. Several goods and methods were tried with no success. Prior to DMSO, organ preservation required the creation of ice crystals, which destroyed the tissue.

Dr. Jacob and Robert Herschler initially met in 1961, and Dr. Jacob learned about DMSO's anti-freeze properties. DMSO is still used for the preservation of transplant organs, among other applications. While 100% DMSO will freeze at 66 degrees, a 50% combination of DMSO and water will not freeze at temperatures far lower than the freezing point of pure water.

Dr. Jacob quickly realized that DMSO has several other qualities that would subsequently make it one of the most important medicinal compounds ever discovered. Just a couple of these features, or perhaps one alone, might make DMSO a valuable substance in the treatment of a wide range of illnesses. When all of these traits are united in a single chemical, we get a truly wonderful result.

Dr. Jacob defined DMSO as a novel medicinal theory. It is a material that is completely unfamiliar to medical science. Its mechanism of action is not fully known, but it is utilized to cure several conditions that were previously thought to be incurable. Furthermore, doing double-masked trials with DMSO is quite difficult due to its unique odor.

However, it is always feasible to conduct experiments with DMSO and compare the findings to current therapy. For example, suppose a disease at a specific stage has an estimated fatality rate of 80% within one year and a 10% mortality rate for those treated with DMSO. In that case, this indicates that DMSO is an effective treatment. If the mortality rate remains at 80%, there is no improvement.

Methylsulfonylmethane, or MSM, is a compound generated from DMSO. MSM contains many of the same qualities as DMSO but is mostly used as a dietary supplement. It has not been studied in the same way as DMSO has, and it is not thought to be as useful in treating most disorders. However, it does not give the patient garlic-like DMSO breath.

DMSO is one of the most effective free radical scavengers known. Free radicals are unstable charged molecular fragments that attack other molecules and cause extensive damage to cells throughout the body. It interferes with the regular functioning of many organs in the body. Free radical damage is generally gradual and builds over time. Cancer and arthritis are two conditions that might result from this over time. It can also contribute to premature aging. It is feasible that consistent usage of DMSO will totally prevent some severe illnesses.

Another key impact of DMSO is normalizing the immunological system. This makes DMSO useful in the treatment of autoimmune illnesses, as well as in assisting the natural immune system in fighting off a variety of infectious and dangerous diseases.

DMSO also permeates the skin and other cellular membranes in the body. This is why applying a modest dose of DMSO topically to the skin can result in a garlic-like breath odor. DMSO is one of the few compounds that can cross the blood-brain barrier. It can also transport other things that would not ordinarily penetrate this barrier. This might make

DMSO useful in the treatment of a variety of brain conditions.

Another key function of DMSO is as a vasodilator. It can enhance blood flow, making it easier to reach places where damage has occurred. An injury frequently results in reduced blood flow to the injury site, and part of the effect is caused by a lack of blood to the region following the injury rather than the injury itself.

On many occasions, DMSO is utilized to address one disease but ends up benefiting another entirely unrelated health concern. It is hoped that this book will encourage more doctors in the United States and other countries to use DMSO, particularly in the treatment of more severe situations where nothing else appears to work.

Why DMSO Remains a Hidden Gem

Imagine discovering a natural substance that has been confirmed to have great therapeutic qualities but is generally unknown and neglected. That is the story of DMSO (dimethyl sulfoxide). Despite its enormous promise, DMSO has remained in the shadows, and many people wonder why it has not received the acclaim it deserves.

The explanation is a combination of bad timing, regulatory prudence, and financial interests that need to be fully aligned with the public good. The history of DMSO, from discovery to current controversy, is an intriguing story.

Back in the 1960s, DMSO held considerable promise as a safe and efficient therapy for a variety of ailments. It was natural, functioned well, and was reasonably priced—almost too wonderful to be true. However, one bad piece of research knocked everything off track. In this study, laboratory animals were given incredibly large doses of DMSO, much above what any human would ever consume, and some of these animals suffered clouding of the lens in their eyes. Naturally, this raised red flags.

However, it is generally ignored that once the DMSO was stopped, many of the animals' lenses cleared up completely. But by then, the harm had been done; DMSO's fate was determined. On November 25, 1965, the FDA issued a ban on all human applications of DMSO.

Why was the decision so severe and rushed? Some feel it was because the FDA was still dealing with the thalidomide debacle. Thalidomide, a medicine intended to relieve morning sickness, resulted in serious birth abnormalities in thousands of infants. The public was outraged, and the FDA was under enormous pressure to avoid another crisis. With this in mind, they may have been too careful when DMSO was under review.

There is also the question of money. DMSO is a natural substance hence no pharmaceutical firm can patent it. Without a patent, there is no significant financial benefit. Dr. Stanley Jacob, known as the "father of DMSO," was allegedly told by a prominent pharmaceutical executive, "I don't care if DMSO is the major drug of our century, and we all know it is. It isn't worth it to us." The truth is that pharma corporations are not interested in marketing a treatment that they cannot benefit from, no matter how successful it is.

Even FDA authorities have confirmed that DMSO is safe. J. Richard Crout, former head of the FDA's Bureau of Drugs, once said that "DMSO is a low toxicity and safe compound." However, he also noted that drug corporations would only invest in something once they perceive a profit.

So, where does this leave us? Despite the setbacks, DMSO is still available, just not in the way you may anticipate. It is marketed as an industrial solvent and is utilized in veterinary treatment, notably with horses. The irony is that while it has been authorized for animal usage, it is still not commonly recognized for human use, except in very rare instances.

DMSO remains the people's medication, a hidden gem that is both accessible and inexpensive. It is up to us to spread this knowledge, use DMSO in our daily lives, and advocate for more access to it. This isn't just about one chemical; it's about our freedom to prefer natural, effective remedies over possibly hazardous prescription medications. In a world where our healthcare options are continuously being curtailed, advocating for our health freedom is more crucial than ever.

So, if you've ever felt like the healthcare system isn't providing you with all of your alternatives, consider DMSO. It's more than simply healing; it's about taking charge of your health and making educated decisions. The more people learn about DMSO, the harder it will be to keep it hidden.

How DMSO Works: Breaking Down the Science

DMSO may sound like something out of a science lab, but it's actually a fascinating substance that functions in some unusual ways. Let us break things down so it is easier to grasp.

At its heart, DMSO (dimethyl sulfoxide) is a byproduct of wood processing, especially papermaking. It is a simple chemical consisting of two methyl groups, one sulfur atom, and one oxygen atom. What distinguishes DMSO is how it interacts with the cells in our body.

Think of DMSO as a highly helpful delivery person. It may easily travel through skin, tissue, and cell membranes, transporting other chemicals with it. This capacity to penetrate so deeply is one of the primary reasons why DMSO is so helpful in treating a variety of illnesses. Once within the body, DMSO begins to act, lowering inflammation, relieving pain, and even assisting in the transportation of other drugs to where they are most needed.

But DMSO isn't just a one-trick pony. It also serves as a potent antioxidant. This implies it helps to neutralize dangerous free radicals, which are chemicals that may injure cells and lead to aging and illness. By absorbing free radicals, DMSO helps to protect cells and keep them running properly.

Another fascinating property of DMSO is its ability to reduce swelling and inflammation. When you apply DMSO to an injury, it helps to pull water out of the tissues, reducing swelling. This is why athletes frequently rely on DMSO for speedy treatment of sprains and strains—it goes to the site of the problem and begins acting nearly quickly.

In a nutshell, DMSO works by entering deep into tissues, lowering inflammation, and protecting cells from harm. It's similar to having a multi-tool in your medical cabinet that can treat a variety of illnesses, from mild pains to major diseases.

The Power of Penetration

One of the most remarkable aspects of DMSO is its ability to pass through your skin and reach the exact location where it is required. The capacity to penetrate deeply is what distinguishes DMSO from other therapies.

Let us break it down. When you have a painful muscle or joint, most lotions and ointments you apply to your skin won't go far. They may soothe the surface, but they do not penetrate deeply enough to treat the underlying issue. DMSO is different. It doesn't simply sit on the surface of your skin; it penetrates the layers, into your muscles, and even into your circulation. This implies that it can provide relief directly to the root of your pain or inflammation.

However, DMSO has more tricks up its sleeve than just that. It can also transport other things as it travels through your skin. Consider combining DMSO with a pain relief cream. The DMSO serves as a shuttle, allowing the active chemicals in the cream to permeate deeper into your tissues. This increases the treatment's effectiveness by delivering it to the areas of your body that require it the most.

One of the reasons why DMSO is commonly used in conjunction with pharmaceuticals is its capacity to transport other chemicals. It can help such drugs operate better by ensuring they reach the correct location in your body. So, whether you're utilizing DMSO for something as basic as pain alleviation or for more complicated diseases, its deep-penetrating strength is a major reason it works so well.

And it's not only about pain and inflammation. DMSO may also trade places with water molecules, making it simpler to pass through your skin. It can also alter the pores of your skin, allowing it and whatever it is carrying to flow through more readily. At greater doses, DMSO can cause the fat molecules in your cell membranes to become more fluid, allowing it to sink deeper into your tissues.

Precautions and Considerations

DMSO (Dimethyl Sulfoxide) is an extremely flexible and strong molecule, but like any tool, it must be utilized carefully to get the maximum benefits while limiting any hazards. Understanding how to incorporate DMSO properly into daily routine is critical, whether you're using it to relieve pain, reduce inflammation, or treat more complicated health conditions. Let's go into the dos and don'ts of DMSO usage, from selecting the appropriate dose to avoiding any adverse effects.

When and Why to Use Different Strengths?

DMSO comes in a variety of doses, each tailored to certain demands and degrees of experience. Here's a full description of when and why you might choose a particular strength.

70-90% Concentration (The Powerhouse)

This is the highest concentration available and is often used in circumstances requiring the greatest potential effect. If you have persistent pain, significant inflammation, or obstinate illnesses that have not responded well to previous therapies, this concentration can be quite beneficial. However, with great power comes great responsibility.

Because it is so strong, this concentration may cause more skin irritation. When you use it, you may experience redness, burning, or tingling sensations. That is why it should be used with caution—apply sparingly and avoid big portions of your skin. If you're new to DMSO, it's best to start with a lesser dosage and only increase to this level if required, and your skin can handle it.

50-70% Concentration (The Middle Ground).

For most persons and circumstances, a concentration of 50-70% is optimal. It is potent enough to penetrate deeply and relieve joint pain, muscular stiffness, and acute injuries such as sprains, yet it is less prone to cause skin irritation than greater doses.

This range is frequently the go-to for everyday use. It is useful for treating parts of the body that require considerable relief while avoiding the increased risk of irritation associated with harsher formulations. If you've already used DMSO and your skin tolerates it well, this dose is an excellent choice for frequent usage.

25-50% concentration (the gentle approach)

If you have sensitive skin or are using DMSO on a sensitive part of your body, a 25-50% dosage is probably your best option. This lower dose is also appropriate for people who are new to DMSO or want to address minor ailments without causing skin irritation.

Because it is milder, this concentration is commonly utilized in applications that do not need deep tissue penetration. It's ideal for treating mild pains, skin issues, and general health applications such as skincare. If you are concerned about potential irritation or are just starting off, this is a safe and effective concentration to use.

Below 25% concentration (The Skin-Friendly Option)

Concentrations of less than 25% are commonly utilized for cosmetic or extremely light applications. This concentration of DMSO is widely used in cosmetic products to improve the absorption of other therapeutic substances. It's soft enough that even individuals with the most sensitive skin may often use it without issue.

These low dosages are great for improving skin health, treating minor skin concerns, and increasing the efficacy of your favorite lotions and creams. They provide all of the benefits of DMSO's transdermal properties while reducing the risk of discomfort.

Potential side effects and how to avoid them.

Even while DMSO is usually considered safe, it can have certain possible negative effects. The good news is that most of these may be readily controlled or totally prevented with a few simple measures. Let's look at the most prevalent side effects and how to avoid them.

Skin irritation is the most common side effect.

The most common complaint among DMSO users is skin discomfort. This might cause redness, irritation, or a burning feeling where you've administered the DMSO. Higher concentrations seem to increase the frequency and severity of irritation.

To avoid this, start with a lesser dose if you're new to DMSO or applying it to a new part of your body. To determine how your skin will react, apply a small quantity to a discrete area of skin and wait 24 hours. If you encounter discomfort, dilute the DMSO with water or a soothing carrier, such as aloe Vera gel, before trying again.

Garlic-Like Odor: A Quirky Side Effect

One of the odd side effects of DMSO is the garlic-like stench it can leave on your breath and skin. It occurs when DMSO is taken into your body and subsequently digested, creating a sulfur molecule that smells similar to garlic. While this side effect is not harmful, it can be unpleasant.

Unfortunately, there is no foolproof way to avoid this odor, but you may reduce it by using lower quantities of DMSO and ensuring adequate ventilation during application. Some people notice that the stench dissipates over time as their bodies adjust to the chemical.

Dry skin: A manageable issue.

DMSO has a drying impact on the skin, especially at high dosages. This might make your skin feel tight, flaky, or irritating, particularly if you use it regularly.

To address this, apply a high-quality moisturizer after using DMSO. DMSO can also be used with skin-friendly oils such as coconut, olive, or jojoba oil to keep your skin moisturized while still benefiting from its qualities.

Other considerations include allergies and sensitivities.

It's also worth mentioning that some people are concerned about allergic reactions to DMSO, especially if they're allergic to sulfur-containing substances. However, DMSO is a distinct molecule from sulfites, sulfa medicines, and other sulfur-containing compounds, and real allergies to DMSO are extremely rare.

If you have a history of allergies, particularly to sulfur-containing medicines, proceed with caution. Again, start with a low concentration and perform a patch test to ensure there are no adverse responses.

Safe Procedures for Internal and External Use

DMSO is a versatile drug that may be used both topically (on the skin) and internally (ingested or administered orally). However, how you utilize it has a big impact on its safety and efficacy. Let's look at some recommended practices for internal and external use.

External Use: Guidelines for Safe Application

When putting DMSO on your skin, hygiene is essential. DMSO is a strong transporter, which means it may attract both good and negative things into your body. Before using DMSO, ensure that the region is adequately clean and free of dirt, oils, and other contaminants. A simple wash in mild soap and water should suffice.

Apply DMSO with a clean cotton pad, cloth, or your fingers (which have been carefully cleansed first). After application, do not cover the area with plastic wrap, tight clothes, or anything else that might trap the DMSO against your skin and create discomfort. Allow the DMSO to soak naturally before applying a moisturizer as needed.

Internal Use: Proceed With Caution.

Some individuals opt to take DMSO internally, but this should be done with a higher level of care. First and foremost, only use pharmaceutical-grade DMSO if you intend to consume it. Lower grades may contain contaminants that are OK for exterior usage but not for internal intake.

Begin internal usage with a very tiny dose—no more than a few drops diluted in water. Pay close attention to your body's reactions. If you suffer any pain, stop immediately and seek a medical practitioner. Internal use of DMSO is uncommon and should always be done with caution and under the supervision of a qualified practitioner.

General Safety Tips.

Stay Informed: Always learn about DMSO before using it. Read up about its advantages, disadvantages, and proper usage.

Listen to Your Body: If anything doesn't feel right, discontinue using DMSO and reevaluate. It's best to be cautious and safe.

Consult a professional. Talking to a healthcare expert, especially if you have pre-existing conditions or are using DMSO internally, can assist ensure you utilize it safely.

Choosing the Right Grade of DMSO: What You Should Know

If you're thinking about utilizing DMSO for health reasons, you should be aware of the many grades available. DMSO is available in two forms: pharmaceutical and industrial grade. While they may appear identical at first appearance, they perform fundamentally different functions—and only one is suitable for human and animal usage.

What's the difference between pharmaceutical and industrial grades?

Let us start with pharmaceutical-grade DMSO. This is the gold standard, with 99.995% purity. That is exceedingly pure, and it is produced by running activated charcoal through the DMSO during the last filtering phase to remove any remaining impurities. This level of purity is what makes pharmaceutical-grade DMSO suitable for usage in humans and animals. So, if you intend to use DMSO for health-related objectives, this is the only grade to consider.

However, industrial-grade DMSO is another thing. This version is not designed for human use, and it usually comes with an explicit warning about that. It is employed in a variety of sectors, including paint stripping, polymer manufacturing, and even agriculture, to help synthesize components such as plant antifungals. Because it is not filtered to the same high standards as pharmaceutical-grade DMSO, it may include contaminants that are dangerous if applied to the skin or swallowed. If you are unclear about the purity of a DMSO product, contact the manufacturer directly for confirmation.

Pharmaceutical-Grade DMSO in Healthcare

Despite some issues along the road with regulatory organizations such as the FDA, pharmaceutical-grade DMSO has established a vital niche in healthcare. It is not as extensively utilized as some other compounds, but when used correctly, it shines. One of its principal functions is as an excipient, which means it serves as a carrier or stabilizer in a variety of medical compositions. DMSO is wonderful for dissolving compounds that are notoriously tough to work with—think stubborn fats, minerals, vitamins, and so on. Furthermore, it accomplishes all of this without causing damage to the fragile structure of these materials.

One fascinating application of pharmaceutical-grade DMSO is organ transplants. Here's how it works: when organs are taken for transplant, they're placed on ice to keep them safe until they're implanted into the recipient. DMSO is given to protect the cells from freezing-related damage. This protective characteristic applies to other medical circumstances as well. For example, some experts believe that DMSO might help lessen the negative effects of some medications or even post-operative issues such as radiation damage.

The Versatility of DMSO: A Carrier of Health

One of the most fascinating aspects of DMSO is its potential to combine with other chemicals. DMSO has a unique potential to increase the absorption of whatever it is combined with, whether it be a prescription, a vitamin, or a natural treatment. This means that DMSO may transport these compounds through the skin, into the circulation, and even across the blood-brain barrier—a notoriously difficult nut to crack in medicine.

The possibilities are practically unlimited. Imagine being able to deliver a critical medication straight to where it is most needed, skipping the digestive system totally. Alternatively, consider taking DMSO to help your body absorb essential nutrients more effectively. It's no surprise that DMSO has such a promising future in healthcare and wellbeing. The possibilities for combining DMSO with other chemicals are endless, and the ability to improve absorption might alter how we approach many home therapies.

DMSO in Daily Life: Foods and Beyond

Interestingly, DMSO is not just available in a bottle at the health store; it is also found in many ordinary foods and drinks. You're probably already ingesting small amounts of DMSO without realizing it. It occurs naturally in foods such as tea, coffee, wine, asparagus, clams, tomatoes, and cooked corn. It has also been found in spearmint oil, nonfat dried milk, barley malt, and natural water. So, DMSO isn't simply a lab product; it's a material we're all familiar with from our meals.

Even our bodies create and release small quantities of DMSO, especially in urine. This implies that tiny levels of DMSO may be passed on to the fetus or kid during pregnancy and nursing, although these amounts are typically extremely small and part of the normal metabolic process.

Healing with DMSO: From Aches to Z

DMSO is like a Swiss Army knife for health—it's extremely versatile and can be used to treat a variety of ailments. Whether you have arthritis, muscular discomfort, skin concerns, or chronic pain, DMSO is a natural and effective remedy. Let's take a step-by-step look at how to employ this strong substance to get relief.

Arthritis Relief: Step-by-Step Guide

Arthritis may be quite painful. Everyday tasks might become difficult when your joints are always aching and constrained. However, DMSO has been demonstrated to provide substantial relief for people living with arthritis.

Here's how to use DMSO to treat arthritis pain:

Begin with Clean Skin: Before using DMSO, ensure that the area you're treating is clean and dry. It ensures that the DMSO penetrates the skin without bringing any unwanted substances with it.

Choose the Right Concentration: For arthritis, a 70% DMSO solution is commonly recommended. This concentration is strong enough to penetrate deeply while remaining gentle on the skin.

Apply gently: Apply a thin layer of DMSO to the affected joint with a clean cotton pad or your fingertips. Be gentle—there is no need to rub it in aggressively. The DMSO will do the task on its own.

Allow It to Absorb: Let the DMSO absorb into your skin. You may experience a slight warming sensation, which is normal. Allow it to work its magic for approximately 20 minutes.

Repeat as needed: You can use DMSO up to three times per day for continuous relief. Monitor your skin for any signs of irritation and adjust the concentration as required.

Many patients discover that their arthritis pain gradually subsides, allowing them to move more freely and comfortably.

Shoulder Pains and Muscle Strains: Specific Applications

We've all been there: overdoing it at the gym, sleeping in an awkward position, or lifting something too heavy. The result? Sore shoulders or strained muscles that make it harder to go about your day. Here's where DMSO comes in handy.

Identify the Pain Point: Pinpoint precisely where the pain originates. DMSO works best when administered directly to the cause of the discomfort.

Use a Lower Concentration: For muscular strains and shoulder discomfort, a 50-60% DMSO solution is generally adequate. This concentration is strong enough to alleviate pain while avoiding skin irritation.

Massage It In: Place a small amount of DMSO on the affected area and gently massage it into the skin. This not only allows the DMSO to penetrate deeper but also increases blood flow to the area, resulting in faster healing.

Pair with Essential Oils: If you prefer, you may mix DMSO with a few drops of essential oils like lavender or eucalyptus. These oils have their pain-relieving characteristics and can improve the calming effects of DMSO.

Rest and recover: After administering DMSO, allow your muscles some time to recuperate. Avoid overexerting the affected area, and you should begin to feel better within a few hours.

Using DMSO can reduce recovery time and allow you to resume normal activities quickly.

Skin Conditions: Eczema, Rashes, and More

Skin problems can be extremely frustrating. Whether its eczema, a persistent rash, or another condition, it can feel like nothing works. However, DMSO has shown promise in treating a variety of skin problems.

Patch Test First: Before applying DMSO to a large area, do a patch test on a small section of your skin. This helps to ensure that you are not sensitive to DMSO.

Use a Diluted Solution: For skin problems, a 30-50% DMSO solution is often advised. This lesser concentration is gentler on the skin yet equally effective.

Apply carefully: Using a clean cotton ball or pad, dab the DMSO solution over the afflicted region. You do not need to saturate the area; a little goes a long way.

Combine with Moisturizers: Because DMSO can be drying, it's a good idea to use a natural moisturizer like aloe Vera or coconut oil afterward. This keeps your skin moisturized and soothes any irritation.

Monitor Progress: Keep an eye on how your skin responds. Some people get results within a few days, while others may take a little longer. Maintain consistency.

DMSO's ability to penetrate deeply into the skin makes it a good choice for treating problems that have proven resistant to conventional therapies.

Chronic Pain Management: Effective, Non-Addictive Solutions

Chronic pain is tiring. It drags you down day after day, and many standard painkillers have a slew of negative side effects and the potential for addiction. DMSO is a natural option that might provide comfort without drawbacks.

Start with a Consultation: If you have chronic pain, you should speak with a healthcare expert before beginning any new treatment, including DMSO. They can advise you on the best approach for your scenario.

Experiment with Concentrations: Because chronic pain differs from person to person, you may need to try several DMSO concentrations to see which one works best for you. Many people find that a 70-90% solution is the most beneficial for severe, ongoing pain.

Apply Consistently: Consistency is essential when using DMSO to manage chronic pain. Apply it on a regular basis to the regions of your body that are most painful, and allow it to work. You may not see effects right away, but many patients see a steady reduction in discomfort over time.

Consider Combining with Other Treatments: DMSO can be used in conjunction with other pain-management measures such as physical therapy, acupuncture, or even medications. Because it helps transport chemicals deeper into the body, it can improve the efficacy of various treatments.

Keep track of your pain levels and how they change after using DMSO. It allows you to fine-tune your treatment plan and make changes as needed.

For people suffering from chronic pain, DMSO is a natural, non-addictive alternative to relieve discomfort and enhance quality of life.

Shield against the Invisible

Radiation is a part of our daily lives, whether we're flying on an airplane, obtaining medical scans, or simply going outside in the sun. But the fact is that radiation is like an unseen enemy—it may enter our cells and inflict harm without us ever noticing it. This is where DMSO (dimethyl sulfoxide) comes in as a possible hero.

When it comes to shielding our cells from the harmful effects of radiation, DMSO has some very astonishing properties. It's similar to arming your body with a shield before entering a combat zone. The magic of DMSO is its capacity to raise glutathione levels, a potent antioxidant that helps shield our cells from the harmful free radicals that radiation produces. These free radicals may damage our DNA, causing aging, illnesses, and even cancer. By increasing glutathione levels, DMSO aids our systems in fighting free radicals, keeping our cells—and ourselves—healthier.

However, DMSO does more than prevention. If you've previously been exposed to radiation, such as through a CT scan or an X-ray, DMSO can still assist. It has been found to accelerate the repair of DNA damaged by radiation. So, whether you're ready for a flight or want to be on the safe side following a medical treatment, DMSO might be your go-to partner in a world where radiation is always present.

Protecting Against Ionic Radiation

We've all heard about the dangers of radiation, whether from medical procedures like CT scans or even from spending time at high altitudes during flights. This type of radiation, called ionizing radiation, has the power to break down chemical bonds and wreak havoc on our DNA. But how exactly does DMSO step in to shield us from this hidden menace?

Let's first look at what happens when our bodies are exposed to ionizing radiation. This type of radiation interacts with our cells and triggers the production of free radicals. Free radicals are unstable molecules that cause widespread damage to proteins, cell membranes, and most critically, DNA. The aftermath of this damage can lead to severe consequences like premature aging and even cancer.

DMSO steps in like a cellular guardian. One of its standout roles is neutralizing these free radicals before they can inflict serious damage. It does this by boosting the levels of glutathione, which is a powerful antioxidant in our bodies. Think of glutathione as the cleanup crew, mopping up free radicals and offering a protective barrier for our cells. When the levels of glutathione are higher, our cells become more resilient against the harmful effects of radiation.

But DMSO's role doesn't end there. It also plays a part in healing previous damage. Studies have shown that DMSO accelerates the repair of DNA strands harmed by radiation. This is vital because damaged DNA can lead to mutations, which, in turn, may cause cells to multiply uncontrollably—one of the key signs of cancer development.

So, whether you're a frequent flyer, work in an environment with high radiation exposure, or are preparing for a medical scan, DMSO offers scientifically backed protection to help minimize the risks.

Versatile Protector and Healer

How to Use DMSO Before and After Exposure

In today's world, radiation exposure is difficult to avoid. We are routinely exposed to small quantities of radiation, whether through medical procedures such as CT scans and mammograms or just flying in an airplane. While these exposures are typically deemed harmless, they can cause some damage to our cells over time. Fortunately, DMSO provides a method for reducing this damage, and taking it adequately can make all the difference.

Before exposure

If you know you'll be exposed to radiation, such as during a CT scan or a lengthy trip, DMSO can help protect your body beforehand. Here's an easy method to utilize it:

Drink the DMSO solution: Mix 1 teaspoon of pure 99.995% DMSO with 5 ounces of distilled water or juice. Drink once a day starting three days before your exposure. This will strengthen your body's natural defenses against the damaging effects of radiation.

After Exposure

If you've previously been exposed to radiation, don't be concerned—DMSO can still help cure the damage:

Topical Application: If you've had a high-exposure procedure, such as a full-body CT scan, try applying DMSO straight to your skin. Apply an 80% DMSO solution to your body as soon as possible after exposure.

Drink a DMSO Solution: As you would before exposure, combine 1 ounce of pure DMSO with 1 ounce of distilled water or juice and drink twice a day. Continue for at least seven days. This helps to drain out the free radicals produced by the radiation, reducing damage and encouraging recovery.

Using DMSO in these ways is like giving your body an advantage in the struggle against radiation damage. It's a simple yet effective way to safeguard your health in today's radiation-filled world.

DMSO as a Lifelong Companion in a Toxic Environment

We live in a toxic world, from the air we breathe to the food we eat and the water we drink. It's almost impossible to avoid them completely, but we may take precautions to safeguard our bodies from their adverse effects. DMSO is one such protection, and it's worth considering as a lifetime friend in our increasingly hazardous environment.

DMSO has the unique capacity to bind to poisons, heavy metals, and other toxic compounds, aiding in their removal from our systems. This is especially crucial since many of these poisons can accumulate over time, resulting in chronic health issues. Heavy metals, such as mercury, lead, and cadmium, can build in our tissues and harm our brain system, kidneys, and other organs. DMSO helps by adhering to these metals and eliminating them from our bodies via urine and sweat.

But DMSO isn't merely for detoxification. It also helps the body's natural healing processes. It increases blood flow, decreases inflammation, and improves oxygen supply to our cells—all of which are critical for staying healthy in a toxic world.

In addition, DMSO is a strong antioxidant. It aids in neutralizing free radicals, which are unstable molecules that can harm cells and contribute to aging and disease. DMSO protects our cells and keeps our bodies running smoothly by keeping free radicals at bay.

Given all of these advantages, incorporating DMSO into your daily routine may be a wise decision for long-term health. Whether you use it locally to treat pain and inflammation, orally to detoxify and guard against radiation, or simply as a preventative step, DMSO is a versatile and efficient strategy to protect your body in a hazardous environment.

Works as an Anti-inflammatory Agent

Inflammation is our body's natural response to injury, yet it may be quite painful. When you're harmed, your body releases a rush of chemicals into the damaged region. This generates redness, heat, swelling, and discomfort, all of which indicate that your immune system is active. However, inflammation can get out of control, causing more harm than benefit. This is where DMSO comes in.

DMSO acts as a natural fire extinguisher for inflammation. It works by inhibiting the release of molecules that induce inflammation, such as prostaglandins and cytokines. DMSO helps to lessen the swelling, redness, and discomfort associated with inflammation.

But DMSO does not end there. It also improves blood flow to the damaged region, bringing in new oxygen and nutrients to hasten the healing process. This is especially critical in chronic inflammation when tissues can become oxygen-starved, resulting in further damage.

In addition to its anti-inflammatory properties, DMSO is an effective pain reliever. It works by inhibiting the nerve signals that transmit pain, delivering comfort without the negative effects of conventional pain drugs.

Whether you have a sprained ankle, a chronic illness such as arthritis, or simply general aches and pains, DMSO is a natural, effective approach to reduce inflammation and get you back on your feet.

DMSO: A Hidden Gem in Cancer Treatment

Most people think of cancer treatment as either chemotherapy, radiation, or surgery. But what if I told you there's another powerful therapy that's been around for over 50 years, yet not many people know about it? It's called DMSO (dimethyl sulfoxide), a remarkable and versatile compound with some seriously promising potential in cancer treatment. What makes it even more intriguing is how well it works when combined with other therapies.

What Makes DMSO Stand Out?

When it comes to how it affects the body, DMSO is pretty special. It acts as a strong free radical scavenger, meaning it helps eliminate harmful chemicals that damage cells and contribute to cancer development. Picture free radicals as tiny troublemakers, wreaking havoc and throwing off your body's natural balance. This is where DMSO steps in—it sweeps these troublemakers out, helping to protect your cells from harm.

But there's more. DMSO is also known for its detoxifying properties, almost like a cleaning crew for your body's cells, clearing out toxins that don't belong. What's particularly unique is DMSO's ability to penetrate biological tissues and target specific cells, making it a perfect delivery system. It can carry other medications directly to where they're needed most, making those treatments more effective. While DMSO has its anti-cancer abilities, it becomes even more powerful when combined with other cancer-fighting drugs.

DMSO's Effect on Leukemia Cells

One of the earliest and most groundbreaking studies on DMSO's anti-cancer properties came from Dr. Charlotte Friend, a leading virologist at Mt. Sinai Hospital in New York City. She wanted to see how DMSO would affect leukaemia cells in the lab. What she found was astonishing: when DMSO was added to leukaemia cells, they began to change. But instead of just slowing down, these cancer cells actually started behaving like healthy, normal cells again. It was almost as if DMSO had pressed a reset button on these cells that had gone rogue.

This discovery was huge because it showed that DMSO could potentially reverse the very process that makes cancer cells so dangerous. Imagine having a tool that could tell cancer cells, "Wait a minute, this isn't right—go back to being normal." That's essentially what DMSO seemed to do in this study.

The Powerful Combo

DMSO and Cyclophosphamide

Cyclophosphamide is an established chemotherapy medication used to treat a variety of malignancies. While indisputably successful, it has major drawbacks. One of the most serious issues is the effect on the immune system. Cyclophosphamide reduces white blood cell numbers, making patients susceptible to infections. This adverse effect is potentially fatal at large dosages.

However, researchers at Nova University in Fort Lauderdale, Florida, achieved a significant breakthrough by combining DMSO (dimethyl sulfoxide) with cyclophosphamide. In a study with rats, a modest dosage of cyclophosphamide combined with DMSO was administered by drinking water, and the effects were amazing.

Not only did the combination efficiently treat cancer, but it also maintained white blood cell count, lowering the risk of infection. In several cases, the cancer was entirely gone, and the rats were considered healed.

This result shows that DMSO improves chemotherapeutic efficacy while dramatically lowering toxicity. It's like having all of the benefits of the medication without the negative side effects—a huge gain for people living with cancer.

DMSO and the Immune System: An Important Ally

Cancer frequently weakens the very mechanism designed to shield you—your immune system. This is where DMSO once again demonstrates its strength. DMSO has been shown in studies to increase the immune response against cancer cells. In multiple investigations, some organisms typically detected in cancer patients and suspected to contribute to cancer progression stopped reproducing when DMSO was added.

Simply put, DMSO strengthens your immune system, helping it fight off hazardous intruders more efficiently. It's like adding another layer of resistance to your body's battle against this difficult condition.

Between 1969 and 1971, one of the most major investigations on DMSO and cancer was conducted at the Military Hospital in Santiago, Chile. The research looked at 65 individuals who were considered incurable and had not responded to conventional cancer treatments. Many of them were in excruciating agony and expected to die from their illness.

The researchers treated the patients with a mixture of DMSO, amino acids, and cyclophosphamide. This technique was unusual since the cyclophosphamide was dissolved in DMSO, which significantly lowered the drug's toxicity while increasing its anti-cancer effects.

Instead of delivering dangerously large doses of cyclophosphamide, the doctors chose lesser dosages given daily or every other day. They observed that even at lower dosages when paired with DMSO, the majority of patients were able to achieve remission—without the severe side effects often associated with chemotherapy.

The results were fantastic. Patients with lymphomas had the greatest improvement, with 21 of 22 reaching objective remission. While not all remissions were lasting, and some patients did not survive, the results were significantly better than expected for such severe cases. Out of the 65 patients, 57 had some remission, whether subjective (based on patient feelings) or objective (based on quantifiable symptoms).

Another notable discovery was the effect on pain. Many patients who had previously been reliant on morphine and other opioids were able to discontinue their use throughout the therapy. This is especially important because chemotherapy often causes greater pain, not less.

Hope for the Hopeless.

Let's look at a real-life example that demonstrates DMSO's potential. Andre Desmond was a salesman for one of the biggest Electronic companies in Los Angeles and was diagnosed with lymphosarcoma, a lymphatic system cancer, and his physician gave him a little chance of life. His family had braced for the worst since the prognosis was bleak.

However, the patient learnt about DMSO and asked his doctor whether it might be incorporated into his treatment regimen. The doctor consented to attempt a low-dose chemotherapy program (particularly cyclophosphamide) together with DMSO. Over the course of six weeks, treatment was administered by slow IV infusion four times each week.

The findings were amazing. Within a week, the patient felt better without experiencing the typical adverse effects of chemotherapy. In fact, he reported feeling better than he had in years. By the end of the six-week course, he was stronger and more active, and six years later, he was still alive and well.

This instance demonstrates how DMSO can not only increase the efficacy of cancer therapies but also significantly minimize their terrible side effects, making the procedure much more bearable for patients.

Why DMSO Should be an Important Part of Cancer Treatment

Based on everything we've covered, it's evident that DMSO has great promise in cancer treatment. It is not only beneficial on its own; it also improves the efficacy of other therapies, such as chemotherapy, while lowering their toxicity.

DMSO's potential to increase the favourable benefits of treatment while decreasing the negative side effects makes it a genuine game changer in cancer care.

Imagine going through chemotherapy without experiencing nausea, exhaustion, or discomfort. Consider knowing that although your therapy is treating cancer, it is simultaneously safeguarding your normal cells. This is the potential that DMSO has for cancer patients.

And this is not simply a hypothetical. Real-world situations, such as the Chilean research and the Los Angeles patient, demonstrate that DMSO can have a major impact on treatment outcomes. It's time to seriously examine DMSO as a normal component of cancer treatment procedures, giving patients a higher chance of not just surviving but also thriving during and after therapy.

Radiation Therapy for Cancer: How DMSO Can Help

Scientists have known about DMSO's radioprotective properties for over four decades, making it a logical option to be administered as a protective agent during radiation therapy for cancer patients. Imagine you're going to be exposed to radiation, which is potent yet has a history of causing severe side effects such as radiation burns. Wouldn't you want something that could protect you against those adverse effects while allowing the therapy to work correctly? This is where DMSO comes in.

To put this idea to the test, a research was done in Russia using cervical cancer patients as participants. The findings were reported in the Russian radiology journal Meditsinkskaia Radiological. In this study, 22 women were moisturized topically with DMSO before receiving radiation treatment. A control group of 59 women who got radiation without DMSO was also observed.

What's the outcome? The ladies who took DMSO did not develop the normal radiation burns that others developed. Meanwhile, the control group had typical burns and toxic effects. It's like wearing armour on a battlefield: DMSO served as a protective shield, sparing these ladies from the unpleasant side effects.

Let's fast forward to a woman in Sacramento who is battling lung cancer. This woman happened to be an ardent reader and follower of my blog, where she learned about the efficacy of DMSO. Her doctor advised heavy radiation treatments to both lungs. When she mentioned using DMSO, her doctor wasn't convinced. He was apprehensive that DMSO would interfere with the radiation. But here's the kicker:

according to some research, DMSO not only protects against radiation's damaging effects, but it actually improves radiation's capacity to combat cancer.

Unfortunately, the doctor's warning had severe effects. The woman's lungs were severely burned after completing her radiation therapy. She required oxygen for three months and experienced terrible times when she was unsure if she would live.

She eventually began DMSO therapy, but unfortunately, it was after the fact. She had weekly injections, drank DMSO mixed with juice twice a day, and applied DMSO lotion on her chest. The recovery was quick, but one has to question how much pain could have been prevented if she had utilized DMSO from the start. The Russian investigation implies that she may not have gotten the burns at all.

In another example, a Southern California lady was diagnosed with lung cancer and referred to a radiologist, who recommended high-dose radiation. However, this time, the doctor was aware of the Russian study's findings on the advantages of DMSO. He explained to the woman that while powerful radiation may effectively treat her illness, it also had the potential to seriously damage her lungs. They chose to utilize DMSO as a topical therapy immediately before each radiation session.

The outcome was nothing short of astounding. This woman underwent radiation therapy without any burns or serious adverse effects. Three years later, she is alive, well, and looking forward to many more years of life. Her doctor is convinced that without DMSO, the radiation would have been hazardous, perhaps leading to an entirely different conclusion.

Exploring DMSO for Diabetes Management

If you have diabetes, whether Type 1 or Type 2, you may discover some interesting information regarding DMSO. While it is not an insulin replacement, many patients have found that including DMSO in their regimen might help them regulate their medical condition. Always check with your doctor before making changes to your insulin plan.

DMSO and diabetic neuropathy

Diabetic neuropathy is a difficult task, particularly for people who have had diabetes for an extended period. It is a disorder in which high blood sugar levels damage nerves, causing numbness or discomfort in the feet and legs. I still recall vividly a story of a patient my colleague shared with me about a man she met while on vacation in Santiago who had had diabetes his entire life. By the age of 64, he could barely walk owing to acute neuropathy in his lower legs and feet. He couldn't feel the earth underneath him.

And she suggested DMSO to him. At first, he was reluctant but later gave it a shot. His therapy consisted of applying DMSO topically to his feet and legs twice a day and consuming a teaspoon of DMSO mixed in juice every evening. DMSO, along with a tight diet and an exercise regimen (which he disliked), helped him restore sensation in his feet. Although he still needs insulin, DMSO has allowed him to live more actively.

Saving toes from amputation

In another example, a Ventura, California, engineer faced the prospect of having two toes removed owing to serious circulation issues. The physician warned that postponing surgery may result in losing part of the foot. The engineer was unwilling to give up his toes and went to DMSO. He used it topically on his toes, foot, and legs. His toes improved substantially over time, allowing him to avoid surgery.

Why DMSO Helps

DMSO works by increasing blood flow. It dilates small blood arteries, increasing circulation to the extremities, which is critical for persons with diabetes. Using DMSO daily might be a preventative rather than a remedy to issues. Ideally, incorporating DMSO into diabetes treatment might help avoid significant complications such as amputations.

The DMSO-Laetrile Combination

Since the 1970s, DMSO has been mixed with laetrile to combat cancer. It has been utilized in various ways, including intravenous injections (slow drip and push methods), intramuscular injections, and topical application to malignant sites. Following the initial therapy, patients frequently continue with laetrile pills and oral DMSO.

Dr. Elmer Thomassen made the first formal use of this combo treatment in Newport Beach, California, in 1977. What about the patient? A New York artist has over 30 melanoma tumours all over his body. He was rushed to California, hoping to find a remedy.

Dr. Thomassen started him on a constant slow infusion of DMSO, laetrile, and vitamin C to intensify the cancer treatment. DMSO and laetrile were given topically to his significant tumors. One tumour on his shoulder was particularly stubborn—that was where his cancer began, and even after being medically removed, it had returned with a fury.

What are the results? The considerable shoulder tumor shrunk by about 50%. Unfortunately, the patient did not survive, but given that he was terminal and had only a few days to live when the therapy began, the fact that his pain was relieved and his health improved was viewed as a success. Even the admitting doctor, who had previously given up hope, began to think recovery was feasible after only one week of treatment.

The second recorded instance included a woman nearing death from tongue cancer and a terrible staphylococcus infection. She was so unwell that she couldn't eat. Her brother, a doctor in Pasadena, took her from the hospital and brought her home, praying for a miracle.

They started her on an intravenous solution, including DMSO, laetrile, and vitamin C. The brother wasn't optimistic, stating, "We'll know in a couple of days. If she is still alive after two or three days, it indicates the therapy is effective.

And it did. Only three days later, she was eating soft foods. Three months later, she was leading normally and had gained more than 20 pounds. The most spectacular cure the brother had seen in over 30 years of practice, she continued to use DMSO and laetrile pills for years afterwards. About a decade later, she was still alive and well when I last spoke with her.

In 1979, a 19-year-old lady received terrible news following brain surgery. The doctors were unable to remove all of the tumor and gave her less than six months to live. However, her family refused to lose hope and took her to the Degenerative Disease Medical Center in Las Vegas for therapy with DMSO and laetrile.

For three weeks, she received one gram of DMSO per kilogram of body weight, six grams of laetrile and 25 grams of vitamin C, administered over four hours daily. Following that, she continued with oral DMSO, laetrile pills, and a diet high in natural, raw foods.

Twenty years later, she was still alive and well. Nobody knows what happened to the tumour because no brain scan was performed following the surgery, but the fact that she lived and flourished says eloquently about the treatment's potential.

More recently, a 56-year-old Los Angeles man was battling prostate cancer. What actually bothered him wasn't the disease but the radiation cystitis produced by his cancer therapy. He was bleeding profusely and had previously received many blood transfusions.

Even though the cystitis was the primary issue, his physicians were able to treat both the cystitis and the malignancy simultaneously with the DMSO-laetrile combination. He was given three ounces of DMSO, 25 grams of vitamin C, and six grams of laetrile via an intravenous slow infusion five days a week for five weeks. He also consumed DMSO combined with aloe vera juice every day.

After only three days, the bleeding had subsided dramatically, and two weeks later, it had ceased. Three years later, he felt better than ever and continued his DMSO-aloe routine, which he intended to keep for life.

Carpal tunnel syndrome is a common and irritating issue, particularly for those who work with their hands frequently. It occurs when the median nerve, which regulates sensation and movement in regions of your hand, is crushed or compressed. This compression can produce various symptoms, including numbness, tingling, and even weakness in your hands and fingers. If left untreated, it can result in irreversible nerve damage and muscular weakness.

Carpal tunnel syndrome has traditionally been treated with night splints, cortisone injections, and different anti-inflammatory medicines. When these approaches failed, surgery was sometimes viewed as a last choice. Conversely, surgery carries its own hazards; for some patients, it might exacerbate rather than alleviate their condition.

This is where DMSO, a chemical recognized for its anti-inflammatory qualities, has demonstrated some potential. Some persons who used DMSO after other therapies failed reported considerable results. While MSM (methylsulfonylmethane), a naturally occurring molecule similar to DMSO, has also proved useful, we will concentrate on DMSO here.

DMSO has various possible advantages for carpal tunnel syndrome. First, it reduces inflammation, which is critical since inflammation in the wrist is what first squeezes the median nerve. Unlike some anti-inflammatory medicines, DMSO has minimal adverse side effects. It also enhances blood circulation in the afflicted region, reducing discomfort.

Consider the instance of a man in Los Angeles who was battling with a particularly stubborn issue known as "trigger thumb." His thumb was so stiff that he couldn't move it, and his previous operation had further exacerbated his problem. Desperate for relief, he decided to try DMSO. He used it twice daily on his thumb, fingers, and hand, then up his arm to the elbow. What was the result? He felt better almost immediately, and within only two weeks, his thumb problem was fully healed. He considered himself cured.

So, while DMSO may not be the first thing your doctor offers, it has shown promise in treating many patients with carpal tunnel syndrome, particularly after other therapies have failed.

Unlocking the Potential of DMSO for Brain Health

As people live longer, dementia, particularly Alzheimer's, has become a significant problem. DMSO might be a game changer in this field since it has shown promise in treating many types of dementia. In clinical investigations, DMSO has been proven to promote the maturation of immature brain cells while simultaneously increasing blood flow to the brain.

As we age, our blood circulation might decrease, depriving the brain of oxygen and vital minerals. This deficiency can damage or even kill brain cells. However, DMSO might help prevent this by increasing circulation and strengthening communication between neurons in the brain. This suggests it may help people maintain their mental acuity far into their senior years. I remember a Maternal Family member who lived to reach 101 years old. She firmly believed in DMSO and had been using it for more than 30 years. Even at 101, she exhibited no evidence of cognitive deterioration. Her knowledge of the Bible was unparalleled, and she was more intelligent than many 30-year-olds. While we don't know how much of this was due to DMSO, it's possible that it helped her intellect stay sharp at such an elderly age. This was when I had little knowledge about DMSO.

One of the most promising applications of DMSO is the treatment of Alzheimer's. According to research, DMSO can remove amyloids, proteins that create plaques in the brains of Alzheimer's patients. These amyloid plaques are strongly linked to the formation and progression of Alzheimer's disease, with larger plaques often indicating more severe dementia.

There is a lot of interest in learning how normal proteins in the brain become amyloid, and inflammation is a crucial factor. Professor Jeffrey Kelly of Scripps Research Institute proposes that inflammation may set off a chain reaction that leads to Alzheimer's. He believes inflammation can disturb normal brain cells, causing amyloid beta proteins to misfold and cause issues.

Kelly discovered evidence of a chemical known as atheronals in the brains of Alzheimer's patients. These atheronals, which form when ozone combines with regular body components, appear to help speed up the misfolding of amyloid beta proteins.

Testing this idea will be difficult, but it provides a reasonable explanation for how Alzheimer's disease may begin, possibly years before any symptoms arise.

A research presented at the Fourth International Conference on Alzheimer's disease and Related Disorders investigated the use of DMSO to treat Alzheimer's patients. In this study, 18 individuals with suspected Alzheimer's were treated with DMSO and monitored for nine months. After barely three months, these patients showed significant improvements. By six months, the benefits in memory, focus, and communication had become more prominent. They were less bewildered, and their general cognitive function had improved.

Given these findings, it appears that anyone exhibiting symptoms of Alzheimer's or another kind of dementia may benefit from DMSO therapy.

The sooner treatment begins, the better, particularly in the early stages of the disease. If the condition progresses far too much, it may be difficult, if not impossible, to reverse the harm. For individuals eager to preserve their mental health as they age, starting DMSO even before any indications of impairment might be a sensible decision.

Ear & Hearing Health: A New Approach

Ear problems are prevalent and can affect persons of all ages. Many children suffer from ear infections during the winter, which are occasionally treated by puncturing the eardrum to relieve pressure. This can be unpleasant, but there is good news: DMSO, when combined with an anesthetic, can make the treatment considerably less uncomfortable. It can also be used with antibiotics to treat middle or inner ear infections without the need for surgery.

Take, for example, an Illinois family with six children who frequently had ear infections. Three of the younger children suffered from terrible illnesses and hearing difficulties one winter. Instead of the standard therapies, they explored a novel approach: DMSO. They had instant alleviation after placing drops of a 50% DMSO solution directly into their ears and a more substantial 90% solution around their heads and necks. Their mother maintained the medication at home, keeping the infections at bay for the remainder of the winter.

Let us now discuss tinnitus, a condition in which patients hear annoying noises such as ringing, buzzing, or even music that does not exist. It can be quite upsetting and is frequently accompanied by hearing loss. Prior to the introduction of DMSO, medical options were limited, ranging from surgery to antibiotics, with variable outcomes.

A 1975 research study from Chile presented at the New York Academy of Sciences found good outcomes for tinnitus with DMSO. This research gave 15 individuals with chronic tinnitus a DMSO spray and other treatments. The findings were impressive: nine patients recovered completely, four improved well, and only two had minor residual problems. Additional advantages included headache and sleeplessness reduction and substantial increases in ear temperature, indicating improved blood flow.

In New York City, a clinic succeeded with a different DMSO treatment. Patients utilized 40% DMSO ear drops daily, as well as a 90% DMSO lotion around their ears. Most patients observed a considerable reduction in ear sounds almost immediately, and many experienced total relief within a month. Even individuals who had not previously pointed out ear problems had an improvement in their tinnitus while receiving treatment for other ailments.

DMSO and Its Role in Arthritis

Over 21 million Americans battle with arthritis daily. It can range from minor discomfort to debilitating pain that takes away movement and joy from life. It's no surprise that arthritis is the leading cause of disability in those over 65. Traditional treatments frequently include a mix of pain relievers, but they mask the symptoms without treating the underlying problem. Aspirin, cortisone, and nonsteroidal anti-inflammatory medications (NSAIDs) help alleviate pain, but they come with considerable hazards, particularly when used for an extended period.

NSAIDs, for example, may alleviate pain but come at a cost. They operate by inhibiting enzymes that create inflammatory substances and enzymes that assist in preserving cartilage, the cushion in your joints. So, while your discomfort may subside temporarily, your joints may sustain more damage over time.

This is where more natural methods come into play. Many people have experienced comfort from supplements such as glucosamine sulfate and MSM. These alternatives do not have the same hazards as regular medications and may often successfully relieve pain. Interestingly, research has found that arthritic joints frequently contain low amounts of sulfur, indicating that sulfur deficiency may play a role in osteoarthritis. This might explain why many arthritis patients find relief after bathing in sulfur-rich hot springs.

DMSO (dimethyl sulfoxide) has emerged as an effective treatment for osteoarthritis and rheumatoid arthritis. While some believe that DMSO can give rapid relief, it's crucial to remember that meaningful, lasting improvement takes time. However, DMSO has repeatedly proven to be a successful therapy, whether given topically, injected, or taken orally.

Initially, most arthritis patients utilized DMSO as a topical therapy, administering it directly to their damaged joints. Today, more modern lotions mix DMSO with additional chemicals to increase their efficacy.

So, what makes DMSO so helpful in treating arthritis? First and foremost, it is a powerful pain reliever that lowers muscular spasms surrounding the joints. It also stimulates blood circulation, allowing vital nutrients to reach damaged regions, and delivers sulfur straight to the joints. DMSO also has powerful anti-inflammatory effects, essential for controlling arthritic symptoms.

Most importantly, DMSO functions as a potent free radical scavenger. Free radicals are unstable chemicals that may harm cells and are linked to various degenerative disorders, including arthritis. This notion was validated by research done in Brazil that provided compelling evidence.

The research at the Centro Internacional de Medicina Preventiva in São Paulo featured 30 patients (15 with osteoarthritis and 15 with rheumatoid arthritis). The purpose was to see if DMSO might lower free radical generation while simultaneously alleviating symptoms. The patients were treated with DMSO, B complex vitamins, vitamin C, and magnesium sulfate. After five weeks of twice-weekly treatments and 18 months of monthly treatments, the findings were impressive: a 66% reduction in free radical generation immediately after DMSO therapy and a 52% reduction by the end of the study. Over 85% of osteoarthritis patients and 77% of rheumatoid arthritis patients had considerable improvement, all without standard anti-inflammatory medications.

DMSO's adaptability is one of its advantages. Some physicians propose topical use for localized arthritis, while others advise ingesting it diluted in juice or water. Patients who have been on heavy drugs for years often discover so much comfort from DMSO that they desire to discontinue all other treatments. However, it is critical to talk with your doctor before making any changes to your pharmaceutical regimen, especially if you have been on prescription meds for an extended period. Your doctor can help you safely reduce or eliminate medications, ensuring that your therapy is both effective and safe.

In the fight against arthritis, DMSO provides a potential, natural option that not only relieves symptoms but also targets some of the disease's underlying causes. With its capacity to ease pain, reduce inflammation, and battle free radicals, DMSO might be the answer for individuals seeking long-term comfort.

Boosting Recovery: How DMSO Can Transform Athletic Injury Treatment

Athletic injuries are sometimes viewed as the outcome of an unexpected mishap, such as a sprained ankle from a hard fall or a fractured bone from an extreme tackle. However, many injuries develop gradually, particularly following strenuous exercises or competitions. You may not recall the exact incident that triggered the discomfort, but little, recurrent pressures on your body can accumulate over time.

Consider marathon runners who push their bodies to the maximum. The persistent pressure and strain on their knees, hips, and other joints can cause serious complications. Sometimes, these injuries appear unexpectedly after weeks or months of relatively minor wear and tear.

The progressive accumulation of tension can damage muscle fibers, resulting in scar tissue and adhesions. Intense exercise might be more detrimental than beneficial if the injury is severe. This is especially true for senior athletes, who must exercise with caution.

That's where DMSO (dimethyl sulfoxide) comes in. For more than 50 years, sportsmen have relied on DMSO to heal and prevent injuries. It's very beneficial to use DMSO before and after strenuous exercise or competitions. Why? Because it reduces inflammation and is extremely good at scavenging free radicals, which are unstable chemicals that can cause more damage following an injury.

Let me provide a few instances. In the 1960s, Sam Bell, a track coach, began utilizing DMSO with his athletes. Two of his runners, Morgan Groth and Norm Hoffman, were dealing with long-term ailments. After being treated with DMSO, they were able to resume training and even became national winners that year.

There's also the story of Darrell Horn, a champion long jumper. Horn was seriously wounded and hobbling only days before a crucial Olympic trial. His health improved substantially with DMSO therapy, allowing him to compete—though he missed the Olympic team by a narrow margin.

And let us not forget June Connelley, a blind distance runner who encountered enormous hurdles in the late 1960s. Despite skepticism and physical challenges, she utilized DMSO to treat her ailments and completed a marathon, finishing among the top participants.

DMSO has an influence that goes beyond injury recovery. It could be a game-changer for contact sports like football and boxing. Imagine if players used DMSO after each game or practice to help lessen the harm from repeated knocks and bumps. Even retired athletes with long-term concerns may benefit from DMSO, whether given topically or ingested in various forms.

DMSO is a viable method for managing and recovering from athletic injuries, helping athletes limit downtime and avoid long-term incapacity.

When a person has a significant brain injury, whether from a vehicle accident, a fall, or a workplace accident, therapy can be extremely difficult. These injuries frequently cause nerve damage, edema, restricted blood flow, and oxygen shortages in the brain. This is where DMSO (dimethyl sulfoxide) may make a big difference.

Here's the key: the sooner you begin DMSO therapy, the better the outcome. While some sources say that treatment should begin within four hours, this is a flexible deadline. Starting DMSO treatment as soon as possible after the injury is ideal, but even if a delay occurs, it can still be beneficial.

The most frequent method of administering DMSO for severe brain trauma is via a steady intravenous infusion. Doctors may provide up to five grams per kilogram of body weight for 24 hours, then lower the dose to two or three grams per kilogram daily. The initial dose is often administered more quickly for the first hour to get things started.

DMSO works wonders by rapidly increasing blood flow to the brain, which is critical since insufficient blood flow can cause brain damage or even death. It also helps to remove extra blood and fluid, which can accumulate and squeeze the brain. Consider it a vital assist in reducing edema and ensuring the brain receives the oxygen and nourishment it requires.

One research in Turkey examined ten individuals with serious head injuries and high intracranial pressure. They got DMSO by IV, and the outcomes were promising. Intracranial pressure fell dramatically during the first 30 minutes, and improvements persisted for many days. CT scans proved that brain swelling had diminished, and most patients recovered well within a few months. While not all patients recovered completely, many saw significant improvements in neurological function.

A real-life example demonstrates DMSO's potential. Jessie Yurick, a brilliant 13-year-old, was seriously injured in 1998 when a horse landed on her head. After being unconscious and suffering from significant memory loss for years, she tried DMSO for the first time in 2011. Interestingly, her mental clarity and vitality increased dramatically following the first treatment, demonstrating how beneficial DMSO may be even years after an accident.

Given the favorable outcomes and low side effects, DMSO is a promising treatment for severe brain damage. While additional study is required, the potential to save lives and improve outcomes is promising.

Finding Relief: How DMSO Can Help with Digestive Troubles

Digestive issues can often be tricky to identify and address, leading to frustration for both patients and doctors. Take, for example, the experience of an eight-year-old girl from Guadalupe. She began throwing up after breakfast almost every day—an alarming situation for anyone but especially worrisome for a child her age. After visiting many doctors, it was determined that she had a severe fungal infection that caused a partial blockage in her intestines. Conventional therapy proved ineffective, and surgery appeared to be the only option.

Instead, physicians chose to attempt DMSO as a last resort. They blended half a teaspoon of DMSO with aloe vera and water and administered it to her twice a day. Fortunately, the vomiting subsided after three days. The therapy was stopped after a week, but the symptoms returned. The symptoms disappeared after being resumed and persisted for two more weeks, and the girl was trouble-free for the next 15 years.

This instance demonstrates how DMSO can occasionally provide a remedy when usual approaches fail. But it doesn't stop there. Dr. Aws Salim, a top free radical damage researcher, has done multiple studies demonstrating DMSO's efficacy in treating digestive disorders.

One research looked into whether DMSO may help with stress-induced stomach damage in individuals with pelvic fractures or severe shock. The study included 177 participants, with 57 getting DMSO. The findings were encouraging: fewer patients in the DMSO group suffered stomach injuries than those who did not get it, and the need for emergency surgery was significantly lowered.

In another study, Dr. Salim investigated how DMSO prevented duodenal ulcers from reoccurring. Over a year, 302 individuals received DMSO, allopurinol, cimetidine (a popular ulcer therapy), or a placebo. The results were precise: DMSO plus allopurinol outperformed cimetidine and placebo regarding ulcer relapse prevention, significantly reducing recurrence rates.

Real-world experiences corroborate these findings. Five patients with long-standing duodenal ulcers in New York City were given DMSO and aloe vera juice. All participants reported no ulcer symptoms and improved overall health throughout the year-long trial. This shows that DMSO might be an effective treatment for ulcers and associated disorders.

Misdiagnosis can also result in unneeded problems. A 55-year-old lady experienced significant stomach issues and was misdiagnosed with age-related angiodysplasia. Her actual problem stemmed from long-term aspirin and Coca-Cola consumption. After switching to DMSO and other therapies, she no longer required blood transfusions and improved her general health. This case emphasizes the significance of making an accurate diagnosis and investigating all possible reasons for a patient's ailment.

Soothing Severe Burns: How DMSO Can Help

Burns may be extremely painful and, in severe cases, life-threatening. They can cause infections and significant consequences in addition to skin damage. However, there is some good news when it comes to treating burns: DMSO (Dimethyl Sulfoxide) mixed with aloe Vera has demonstrated exceptional efficiency. Consider an incident from Santa Barbara, California. A restaurant cook had second-degree burns as a result of an accident involving boiling fat. The burn covered a large portion of his body, and the agony was severe. The physicians treated his injuries with a lotion containing 50% DMSO and 50% aloe vera.

The treatment strategy was basic yet effective:

Immediate Relief: The initial application of the lotion was done instantaneously.

Follow-up: An hour later, a second application arrived, and a third three hours later.

Consistent Care: Following the initial treatments, the lotion was used every eight hours for two days.

The findings were remarkable. The cook recovered completely and much faster than predicted with alternative therapies. Not only did the DMSO therapy prevent severe scarring, but it also reduced his recovery period to two days rather than almost a week. The doctor was clear that without the DMSO therapy, the cook would have had considerably more severe problems and a longer recovery time.

However, DMSO is not just used to treat severe burns. It can help treat minor burns, such as those caused by touching a hot pan. DMSO-aloe Vera lotion can help prevent blisters and relieve discomfort. This therapy is effective for sunburns as well. Many clinicians using DMSO for burn therapy believe mixing it with aloe Vera produces the most significant outcomes.

Finding New Hope for Liver Health with DMSO

Cirrhosis of the liver is a dangerous disorder that can result in an excruciating death. Imagine a group of individuals in downtown Los Angeles who have developed liver cirrhosis as a result of extensive drinking, poor eating, and harsh living circumstances. These patients, who were thought to be terminally sick, were given a glimpse of hope after receiving an experimental therapy using DMSO.

To take part in the study, participants had to give up alcohol entirely. Each was given one teaspoon of DMSO along with an ounce of aloe vera juice twice a day, for six months. Of the twelve people involved, only eight made it to the end of the program.

The results were remarkable. These eight individuals saw major improvements in their health. Their nausea and vomiting lessened, liver function tests showed signs of healing, and they reported feeling much better overall. What stood out even more was that, after a year, all eight were still alive and thriving—a future that had seemed nearly impossible before the treatment.

But it's important to make something clear: DMSO was not a magic fix. The patients had to quit drinking and face the consequences of their past habits. While DMSO helped their bodies repair themselves, it wasn't a cure for the damage caused by harmful behaviors.

Why DMSO should be a staple in emergency care.

Let me relate my personal experience with DMSO or dimethyl sulfoxide and explain why I feel it should be included in every emergency room and first aid bag. Having witnessed the benefits of DMSO, it's evident to me that it's an underappreciated resource in emergency medical circumstances.

Years ago, I worked in an industrial medicine clinic in Los Angeles, where we frequently used DMSO on workers who arrived with new injuries. My colleagues and I saw that DMSO may assist in managing various conditions, even if it does not always give an in-depth solution. We frequently began treatment with a topical application of DMSO to the wounded region to avoid additional harm while we evaluated the patient.

One noteworthy incident showed a woman who had a massive stroke and was sent to the emergency hospital in San Gabriel Valley. Her family was enthusiastic about using DMSO in her therapy. Initially, the emergency department doctor was cautious since he had never used DMSO. However, because of the tenacity of a nurse who backed the family's request, DMSO was provided. The following day, a neurosurgeon took over her care and ordered DMSO to be given to her IV, recognizing its potential advantages despite the severity of the injury.

Another startling case from my own experience included a nurse being hit by a vehicle. She was in excruciating pain and concerned about long-term stiffness from the injury. I administered DMSO topically to her body less than 10 minutes after the occurrence and made her swallow a little dose mixed with juice. Within two hours, I had reapplied the DMSO. To my and her astonishment, she felt much better the following day, with minimal discomfort and no stiffness. She was surprised by how well she felt, considerably above her first expectations.

These personal experiences have taught me how useful DMSO can be in emergency situations. Its ability to be administered topically makes it simple and beneficial for many urgent situations. If more individuals, especially medical professionals and first responders knew and used DMSO, emergency treatment may be transformed, dramatically improving patient outcomes in critical situations.

Managing Headaches with DMSO: A Unique Approach

Most of us have had headaches at some point in our lives. Whether it's the steady pulse of stress or the searing agony of a migraine, nearly everyone experiences them at some point. About half of all Americans have at least one headache every month. The causes of severe headaches can be as varied as the pain itself—muscle tightness in the neck, changes in blood vessels, or how our bodies manage stress.

For many, the first line of defence is a short aspirin dosage. But if you've ever experienced a migraine, you know that aspirin isn't necessarily the solution. In reality, it might only make a dent. This is where DMSO, a relatively unknown therapy, comes into play. DMSO has been used to treat headaches for over 40 years, frequently with excellent results and without the side effects associated with many traditional pain drugs.

However, when it comes to migraines, timing is essential. Even DMSO may not be effective while a migraine is in full swing. However, if you detect it early—right when you feel the first twinge—DMSO can occasionally stop the headache in its tracks. DMSO is most commonly used to treat headaches by applying it topically to the head, neck, or both. It can also be consumed orally, combined with juice or water, or injected in rare situations.

I remember a young woman I knew in Newport Beach, California, who had been suffering from progressively terrible headaches for months. They were getting more regular and painful, and they were beginning to disrupt her everyday life. Following various tests, physicians discovered a thin film on her X-ray that they couldn't explain. They decided to try something new and placed her on a DMSO regimen that included topically applying it to her head as well as a modest oral dosage mixed with water.

When she returned ten days later, she stated that her headaches had become worse. The doctor was surprised and questioned whether she had followed the medication as advised. That's when she admitted that, believing "more is better," she had taken four ounces of DMSO instead of the recommended modest quantity, diluting it with a quart of water. Fortunately, DMSO is relatively safe, even at greater dosages, but this was a clear example of why following instructions is critical.

Her headaches began to subside once she returned to the proper dosage of a teaspoon of DMSO in water and topical treatment. Six months later, she was headache-free and never had to return for further treatment.

DMSO can be a game changer for those suffering from chronic headaches, especially if previous therapies have failed. Just remember that, like any therapy, you must follow the instructions and be patient with the procedure. The correct approach can mean all the difference.

Reviving Vision: How DMSO is Changing Eye Health

Eye issues can be challenging to manage, particularly as we become older. However, a surprise ally has recently returned: DMSO (Dimethyl Sulfoxide). Despite a rocky start in the 1960s, when DMSO was restricted owing to worries about eye toxicity in animals, it is now proving to be a game changer for human vision health.

Let's look at how DMSO can assist, particularly for people suffering from significant eye disorders such as retinitis pigmentosa, a leading cause of blindness. Dr. Robert Hill of Longview, Washington, founded DMSO Eye Care. His revolutionary study was featured in the January 1975 New York Academy of Sciences edition.

One famous example included a patient with retinitis pigmentosa who had significantly impaired eyesight. The outcomes of commencing therapy with a 50% DMSO solution given directly to the eye twice a day were outstanding. Five days in, the patient's vision improved dramatically—from seeing only hand gestures to counting fingers from five feet away. By three months, his eyesight had recovered significantly, demonstrating the effectiveness of DMSO in reversing vision loss.

Dr. Hill did not stop there. His study enlarged to include 50 individuals with retinitis pigmentosa or macular degeneration. Out of them, 22 experienced improvement in their eyesight, 9 had better visual fields, and five had improved dark adaption. Only two patients deteriorated, while the others showed no noteworthy changes. Without this medication, these individuals' conditions were sure to worsen.

DMSO offers more than just a glimmer of hope for those struggling with certain health conditions; it has also been applied to treat various eye issues, often with remarkable results—even when the root cause of the problem isn't entirely understood. Some people have reported better vision and reduced discomfort after using DMSO eye drops. Typically, a 40% DMSO solution is used once a day, and while it may cause a brief stinging sensation, that feeling tends to fade quickly, leaving the eyes feeling rejuvenated.

Consider a few real-life success stories. One involves a 90-year-old man who had all but given up on reading due to macular degeneration. His eyesight had deteriorated to the point where reading was no longer possible. However, after a month of applying 40% DMSO eye drops daily, along with taking a teaspoon of DMSO mixed in orange juice, he found himself able to read his favorite books again. His overall health seemed to improve as well, suggesting that the benefits of DMSO could extend beyond just vision improvement.

Another compelling case features a 78-year-old man who had been told by his doctors that nothing could be done to fix his vision problems. Refusing to accept this, he sought a second opinion and began DMSO treatments. His eyesight, which had been 20/200 at the start, improved to 20/100 within two weeks and later progressed to 20/50 with the help of glasses. Over time, his vision stabilized, showcasing DMSO's potential to either halt or even reverse certain types of vision loss.

These stories point to DMSO's promising role in eye health, offering real improvements where other treatments have failed.

Even for ordinary eye tiredness, DMSO eye drops have been effective. Personal use has proven that a 40% DMSO solution will instantly relieve tired eyes, making it an ideal cure for anybody experiencing the strain of a long day.

Harnessing the Power of DMSO for Hair and Scalp Health

DMSO has been a go-to remedy for boosting hair growth for decades, especially in people who have recently experienced hair thinning or loss. If you've just noticed your hair thinning, DMSO could be your best chance. However, if you've been bald for years, DMSO—or any other substance for that matter—is unlikely to restore your complete head of hair miraculously. When hair begins to grow back, it usually appears first in the regions where it was previously gone.

Interestingly, this does not only apply to humans. Animals, such as cats, have demonstrated comparable findings. In other cases, cats who had lost patches of fur totally regrew their hair after being treated with a DMSO-based lotion. Even animals with no hair loss had thicker, healthier fur in the regions where DMSO was administered.

Both men and women who lost their hair following chemotherapy have experienced promising improvements with DMSO. One doctor, who didn't expect such quick hair restoration, recommended his patients to apply DMSO lotion to their scalps. He was shell-shocked, that their hair returned considerably faster than expected, which pleased the patients.

So, why does DMSO promote hair growth? The key lies in its capacity to expand the blood vessels. When applied to the scalp, DMSO dilates the tiny capillaries, allowing more blood and nutrients to enter the hair follicles. This nutritional boost can help restart hair development, especially in male pattern baldness. While progress might be delayed, many people have experienced favourable outcomes.

Speaking from personal experience, I've been using DMSO lotion on my hair for almost ten years. At 45, I still have a full head of natural brown hair. While I can't say for sure that DMSO is the only cause for this,

I feel it has played an essential role in keeping my hair health and colour.

A remarkable instance is about an 80-year-old guy in Oklahoma dealing with a sticky substance dripping from his scalp. After seeking medical attention, he was advised by a doctor that he required surgery to remove a portion of his scalp to address an underlying illness. Understandably, he thought this approach was a little too extreme. Instead, he applied DMSO lotion on his scalp. Six months later, the infection had subsided, and he had a healthy scalp without surgery.

DMSO may not be a miraculous treatment, but it has improved the health of many people's hair and scalp. DMSO should be part of your routine whether you have thinning hair or scalp difficulties.

Fibromyalgia: A Personal Journey of Relief

Fibromyalgia is a complex ailment that might feel like an unsolved conundrum. It is most frequent in women over 50 and mainly affects muscles, tendons, and ligaments. Unlike arthritis, which affects the joints, fibromyalgia causes pain throughout the body. It's difficult to diagnose since its symptoms coincide with many conditions.

Diagnosing fibromyalgia frequently entails coping with extensive pain for more than three months, affecting all four quadrants of the body—both sides, above and below the waist. There is also an exceptional pressure sensitivity, making simple touches uncomfortable. In addition, many patients have bowel and bladder problems and swallowing difficulties and frequently suffer from anxiety or despair.

So, what is the cause? No one knows for sure, but one idea proposes that patients with fibromyalgia may have a reduced pain threshold due to their increased sensitivity to pain signals.

Traditional therapies such as pain relievers, corticosteroids, and antidepressants have not always been effective. However, DMSO and MSM have shown some potential as an alternative strategy.

Combating Fungus Infections: DMSO to the Rescue

Fungus infections, ranging from athlete's foot to tenacious jungle rot, may be an unpleasant experience. Fortunately, DMSO (dimethyl sulfoxide) has demonstrated inspiring results in curing these troublesome issues. Let us look at how it can make a difference.

Jungle Rot and its Remedies

Jungle rot is a tenacious virus that thrives in hot, moist environments. Veterans of World War II and Vietnam who spent time in tropical locations frequently battled this complex illness. One such veteran was Dr. Robert Entin of Los Angeles. After spending a fortune on numerous treatments for his jungle rot, he discovered relief in a skin cream combining DMSO and aloe Vera. While it did not totally cure the illness, it did give great relief when other treatments had failed.

A doctor from the Veterans Administration in Los Angeles later treated additional veterans with the same DMSO lotion. The results were terrific, providing instant relief. However the fungus occasionally returned, particularly during warmer weather. The doctor felt that DMSO lotion was the finest choice available and recommended it to all veterans with fungal infections.

Athlete's Foot and Foot Health

Athlete's foot, a common fungal infection, responds positively to DMSO. DMSO, which is used in dosages ranging from 50% to 90%, can be combined with additional compounds such as capsicum pepper and aloe Vera to increase its efficiency. Typically exacerbated by heated, enclosed shoes, this condition can be efficiently treated with DMSO. Sometimes, it even yields a complete cure. To improve results, let shoes dry completely to eliminate any remaining fungal spores.

Treating Nail Fungus

Fungus under the fingernails and toenails can be very tough. Applying DMSO directly to the affected nail and surrounding skin, generally, twice a day, can help control and frequently eliminate the infection.

Combating Foot Odor

Even when there are no infections, foot odour can be unpleasant. Clean socks and feet help, but they are only sometimes enough. This is where DMSO can come in. Applying it softly to your feet might help to eliminate smells and excess moisture. Long-term treatment may require the use of DMSO daily. One application may provide immediate relief, but frequent usage can keep the stench at bay for an extended time.

My acquaintance used to have persistent athlete's foot, and I recalled him struggling. Despite trying many over-the-counter medicines, he received no relief. He chose to test DMSO after learning about its benefits. He used it religiously, and after a week, he observed a considerable reduction in itching and pain. He was overjoyed to finally discover something that worked and continued to include it in his daily routine.

DMSO provides a diverse solution for controlling and treating different fungal diseases. It's been a tremendous ally, whether it's jungle rot, athlete's foot, or nail fungus. If you're battling persistent infections or unpleasant smells, DMSO might be the remedy you've been looking for.

Infections

Regarding infection control, DMSO has proven to be a game changer, whether taken alone or combined with antibiotics and other treatments.

I'm not a doctor, but based on my observations and experiences, I feel that DMSO should be used as a first-line treatment for severe infections, particularly when conventional antibiotics fail. I recall hearing of a 90-year-old guy in Los Angeles who had a terrible bladder infection that refused to go away despite weeks of medication and other treatments. The physicians were worried if he would survive the disease. As a final option, they decided to incorporate DMSO into his therapy regimen, combining it with cranberry juice. The results were fantastic. The infection had been controlled in just a few days, and the guy was ready to return home. Not only did he overcome the illness, but his overall health and mobility improved.

These examples demonstrate DMSO's effectiveness, particularly when conventional therapies fall short. It's a treatment worth exploring for any severe infection, especially when other alternatives don't work.

Inflammation

Inflammation is the body's natural response to injury or damage. While it is intended to be a healing process, it may occasionally become a more significant problem, particularly when it lasts longer than expected. Consider this: if you've ever twisted your ankle or had a severe burn, you've definitely observed how it swells, becomes hot, and aches. That is your body attempting to restore itself, but when inflammation becomes chronic, as in arthritis, it can cause continual pain and suffering.

This is where DMSO steps in as an unsung hero. This unique compound has demonstrated a great talent for reducing inflammation without the terrible side effects of more typical medications. When patients begin taking DMSO, I've seen swelling reduce before my eyes, the heat of inflammation dissipates, and they instantly experience pain relief. It's like giving your body a helpful hand without the baggage.

Now, let's speak about cortisol, the natural anti-inflammatory hormone. Cortisol, produced by the adrenal glands, is essential for managing inflammation. However, things go out of balance when our systems cannot create enough cortisol or when inflammation gets too severe. Doctors frequently use steroids such as cortisone in this situation. Sure, steroids can save lives in modest amounts. Still, if used for an extended period, they can create a slew of significant problems, including gastrointestinal bleeding, weakened bones, and even mental health difficulties.

Nonsteroidal anti-inflammatory medicines (NSAIDs), such as ibuprofen or aspirin, are also commonly used to treat inflammation. But here's the catch: NSAIDs may be problematic for your stomach and intestines.

Long-term usage can cause ulcers, bleeding, and other digestive issues. Nonetheless, many take these tablets without comprehending the hazards, typically because they are readily available and highly marketed.

This is where DMSO shines. It not only addresses inflammation directly, but it also helps to minimize the adverse side effects of medications such as NSAIDs. Dr. Aws Salim, a world-renowned free radical specialist, did an intriguing study. He tried DMSO on arthritic patients who had acquired major gastrointestinal problems due to long-term NSAID treatment. The results were astounding—patients treated with DMSO saw considerable recovery in their gastrointestinal tracts, far outperforming those not treated.

In fact, a medical facility in Newport Beach, California, has been employing DMSO as the primary treatment for arthritis and injuries. The doctors there saw something remarkable: patients who had significant digestive difficulties due to earlier NSAID and steroid treatments saw their stomach troubles improve dramatically after switching to DMSO. Some people who had been told they would have to live with their agony and bleeding were eventually able to find relief.

Interstitial cystitis

The FDA initially authorized DMSO in 1978 for the treatment of interstitial cystitis, a painful condition in which the bladder's inner lining becomes inflamed. Prior to the discovery of DMSO, there was little hope for patients suffering from this condition because standard therapies such as antibiotics were ineffective. Unlike ordinary cystitis, which is frequently caused by bacteria and may be treated with antibiotics, interstitial cystitis is not caused by bacteria. This made finding an effective therapy challenging until DMSO entered the picture.

For those unfamiliar with the condition, interstitial cystitis may be a nightmare. It can cause significant bladder difficulties such as scarring, bleeding, and a decreased ability to hold urine. The discomfort is typically severe, especially when the bladder is full, and relief is only obtained after urinating. Imagine feeling the need to urinate 50 times every day—that's the reality for some people with this illness, and it doesn't go away when the sun sets. This illness affects hundreds of thousands of people, primarily women.

Initially, DMSO therapy entailed putting a catheter into the bladder to give the solution directly, which was done once or twice a week. However, not everyone could stand the discomfort of this approach. Therefore, an alternative was created: oral DMSO. Many physicians think taking DMSO orally in water or juice is the best option. It is easier, and patients frequently feel almost instant relief. A standard treatment would include a teaspoon of DMSO mixed with cranberry juice, taken once or twice daily. This strategy also eliminates the need for regular medical visits, a significant relief for many people.

Some clinicians prefer a combined approach, beginning with a bladder instillation and progressing to oral DMSO to maintain the treatment's efficacy. This appears to work successfully for many patients.

Both interstitial cystitis and radiation cystitis are severe disorders that can have a significant impact on a person's quality of life. However, DMSO has shown to be a viable treatment choice for both, providing hope where other treatments fail. And, because DMSO is non-toxic, there's minimal danger, even if the diagnosis is uncertain—an essential issue considering how frequently interstitial cystitis is misdiagnosed. DMSO provides alleviation, making it a game changer for anyone suffering from these challenging illnesses.

The Power of DMSO Combinations

DMSO is outstanding on its own, but when coupled with other natural remedies, it may be highly effective. This chapter delves into several lesser-known yet effective combinations that increase the healing potential of DMSO. Before we get into the details, keep in mind that DMSO should not be used with prescription drugs. If you are using any prescribed pharmaceuticals, you should check with a trained physician before beginning any DMSO therapy or making any adjustments to your medication.

DMSO in Black Salve.

Black salve is a mild yet efficient remedy for removing splinters, ticks, glass, insect poison, and even tiny cactus needles from under the skin. What makes it so effective? DMSO is an essential component. It improves the salve's capacity to remove foreign things while minimizing tissue injury. If you're intrigued about black salve, there's a plethora of information available online that you should look into more.

DMSO and Essential Oils

One of DMSO's distinguishing characteristics is its capacity to transfer both water and oil-soluble compounds through the skin. While the amount of molecules it can carry is limited, DMSO can transport essential oils into the body despite their size. In my experience, essential oils are likely to cause a tingling feeling when ingested in this manner, so use caution, especially around youngsters or pregnant and nursing moms.

Essential oils penetrate naturally into the skin, but they are typically combined with a carrier oil, such as sweet almond or grapeseed oil, to prevent irritation and for equal absorption. These oils are volatile, so they evaporate quickly; therefore, combining them with a carrier oil helps prevent loss. Combining essential oils and DMSO increases absorption into the skin and reduces evaporation, making the oils more effective.

Using DMSO as a carrier for essential oils allows you to use less oil to attain the desired result. DMSO sends the essential oil deeper into the tissue, which is very useful for treating deep infections or detoxifying regions such as joints. Toxins will either be dissolved and cleared by the lymphatic system or pushed to the surface for ejection. Suppose you observe any responses, such as a boil forming. In that case, it's typically an indication that the body is mending and eliminating something terrible, not that the therapy is generating a new problem. Using DMSO alone can help avoid subsequent infections and aid the drainage process.

Many individuals misinterpret these reactions as harmful side effects when, in fact, they are part of the body's natural healing process. Understanding how DMSO interacts with essential oils and other medicines allows you to maximize its effectiveness and assist your body's efforts to heal from within.

Exploring essential oil combinations with DMSO

DMSO is already a powerful compound on its own, but when combined with essential oils, it becomes even more potent. In this part, we'll look at several common combinations you may attempt at home, but remember to tread cautiously—especially when utilizing powerful essential oils. Let's look at some of these combinations.

Wintergreen Oil

Wintergreen oil, recognized for its anti-inflammatory and pain-relieving qualities, is frequently used with DMSO. However, this combination necessitates special precautions. 1 or 2 drops of wintergreen oil combined with ten drops of 80% DMSO is generally plenty. Wintergreen oil should be avoided by anybody with liver illness or who is taking aspirin since it contains methyl salicylate, which the liver processes. If you are on blood thinners or have liver issues, you should pick another choice.

Peppermint Oil

Peppermint oil is another popular remedy for headaches and nerve pain, such as sciatica. Rub 1 drop of peppermint oil with 10 drops of 80% DMSO on your temples or the afflicted region for quick relief. This combo is especially beneficial if you are suffering from pain caused by prolonged sitting or managing osteoarthritis. The cooling effect of peppermint and DMSO's deep tissue penetration makes it an ideal combination for reducing inflammation and stress.

Black Pepper Oil

Black pepper oil might be the solution if you suffer from swollen legs or ankle water retention. This warming oil has a beneficial effect on the lymphatic system. Combine 1 or 2 drops of black pepper oil with 10 drops of 80% DMSO and massage into your legs, beginning at the bottom and progressing higher. The interaction of black pepper and DMSO increases blood flow, making this combination helpful in boosting circulation and lowering edema.

Sweet Birch Oil

Sweet birch oil is a natural muscle relaxant that can help relieve tense, stiff muscles. Mix 1 or 2 drops of sweet birch oil (or perhaps clary sage for added relaxation) with 10 drops of 80% DMSO and massage the mixture into your muscles twice a day. This mixture relieves stress and promotes relaxation, making it easier to recuperate after a strenuous workout or a long day.

DMSO and CBD Oil

CBD oil, which is produced from the cannabis plant, is gaining popularity due to its potential to relieve pain and anxiety. When taken with DMSO, the benefits are enhanced, providing a potent option for people seeking comfort without using prescription opioids. While THC, cannabis' psychoactive component, can create hallucinations in large dosages, CBD combined with DMSO concentrates on pain relief and relaxation.

This combination is very good to the neurological system, helping to treat illnesses such as seizures, multiple sclerosis (MS), and even cancer. DMSO improves CBD distribution to cell receptors, resulting in healing processes throughout the body. However, because cannabinoids are fat-soluble and metabolized by the liver, it is critical to support your liver and kidneys when taking CBD with DMSO. Simple measures like staying hydrated and employing liver detox treatments like castor oil packs or topical magnesium chloride can significantly impact how your body manages these substances.

It's also worth mentioning that regular recreational cannabis users may discover that topical or oral CBD is less helpful for pain management owing to THC and CBD saturation in their bodies. This is especially true if they eat processed meals, smoke, or drink alcohol frequently. Over time, the body works to eliminate cannabis waste products, reducing the therapeutic benefits.

In my experience, cannabis-based medicines applied topically or as an extract are more effective and have fewer adverse effects than smoking. However, it is critical to recognize that continuous cannabis usage, particularly before the age of 25, can result in lasting brain damage. Adults can recover from some of the harm after discontinuing usage, but younger users may suffer long-term consequences.

How to Use DMSO with Cannabis Extract

Adding DMSO to cannabis extract can be an effective strategy to boost the effects of CBD and THC. Begin with a high-quality CBD extract, preferably liquid, and combine it with a 50% DMSO solution. This combination can be used to target places where the nervous system absorbs the most effectively. I recommend massaging it on your temples, the back of your neck (just over your spine), and even the soles of your feet after a nice wash. These areas help the body absorb the combination fast.

Begin with around 15 mL of the liquid combination. This quantity is generally sufficient to determine how your body responds. If you feel sleepy the next day, it might indicate that your liver needs more help cleansing. In that scenario, a liver cleanse or just using the combination early in the evening may be precisely what you need.

If you wish to combine THC and CBD with DMSO, choose a cannabis strain that leans significantly toward CBD. When I make this combination, I extract oil from the dried plant in the same way that I would any other medicinal plant. I also prepare a DMSO extract from the dried material, which absorbs the plant's water-soluble components. When these two extracts are mixed, they generate a potent cocktail that can relieve anxiety and immediately provide a sensation of calm. Just be cautious about the dosage—this is powerful medicine, and a little goes a long way.

Combining DMSO and Castor Oil

Castor oil is recognized for its deep-penetrating characteristics, making it an excellent companion to

DMSO, which also penetrates the skin well. When these two mix, the results are nothing short of spectacular.

Castor oil on its own has various advantages. It softens masses, detoxifies organs, and even dissolves calcified deposits in arthritic joints. For detoxification, I usually recommend castor oil packs. You quickly make them at home by soaking a piece of wool flannel or cotton fabric in castor oil and applying it to the problematic region using a heat source such as a hot water bottle. Keep the pack on for about 20 minutes each day, and remember to drink lots of water—at least 8 to 12 glasses each day—to help flush out the toxins.

When you mix DMSO with castor oil, the effects are even more astounding. This combo works wonderfully for rheumatic symptoms, pain, stiffness, and even tendon and joint repair. Many patients have reported quick pain alleviation and decreased scar tissue and other growths. However, this therapy is not appropriate for malignant tumours, and women should avoid taking castor oil during menstruation, pregnancy, or breastfeeding.

How to Use DMSO with Castor Oil?

Begin by applying a slight castor oil coating to the desired treatment region, ensuring the skin is clean and dry. Next, apply an 80% to 90% DMSO solution to the castor oil and let it work for about 10 minutes. Earlier, I said that 80% DMSO should be the maximum dose for home usage. In this situation, the castor oil will naturally dilute the DMSO, lowering the possibility of burning or drying your skin. If you are still concerned about how your skin may respond, use a lesser dosage of DMSO.

Keep in mind that castor oil can stain textiles, so if you treat your feet, make sure to wear clean cotton socks afterwards. Either leave the mixture on your skin or, after 20 to 30 minutes, use a basic baking soda solution to remove the greasy residue. You don't need to add heat because DMSO naturally heats the castor oil, but if you like, lay a hot water bottle wrapped in a tea towel over the region for extra comfort.

DMSO with Colloidal Silver

Colloidal silver is frequently promoted by homoeopathic and naturopathic practitioners as a natural antibiotic that does not add to the issue of antibiotic resistance. It has various strengths and may be used orally as a supplement or applied straight to the skin. When you combine colloidal silver and DMSO, you get a potent combination. DMSO is more than simply a carrier that improves drug absorption into the body's tissues; it also possesses bacteriostatic qualities, which means it can suppress bacterial development. This pair can handle infections, whether they are systemic or localized skin issues.

How to Use DMSO and Colloidal Silver

For anyone wondering how to use this combo, it's actually simple. Begin by combining pure pharmaceutical-grade DMSO with colloidal silver at a concentration of 10 to 15 ppm (parts per million). You should utilize a 50:50 ratio. This mixture may be swished in your mouth as a mouthwash; make sure to spit it out thoroughly when finished. It is ideal for treating oral infections or simply maintaining good oral hygiene.

This same combination may be used topically to treat wounds, whether infected or not, to aid healing. If you have a sinus infection, you can mix it with saline to flush it out. If you have stomach problems such as bacterial overgrowth in the small intestine or ulcers, consider mixing 5 mL of this 50:50 mixture with 2 ounces of distilled water and drinking it. It's a simple yet efficient technique to treat stomach or digestive issues.

DMSO with Botanical Medicine

The purpose of botanical medicine is to extract the plant's medicinal components, also known as constituents, using a solvent. Water is the most used solvent. You may prepare teas (infusions), simmer plants on the stove to generate stronger brews (decoctions), or even allow them to ferment over time. Water will extract the plant's water-soluble components, which are normally very useful.

Another prominent solvent for plants is alcohol, which is used to make tinctures. Alcohol can remove both water and oil-based components, making it a flexible choice. On the other hand, oil-based extractions are generally employed for topical treatments. I've produced numerous skin-healing salves, oils, and creams in this manner, utilizing methods such as heating the oil and herbs on the stove or even letting them sit in the sun for a gradual, UV-assisted extraction.

DMSO, as you might expect, is a good solvent. However, unlike alcohol, DMSO is aprotic, which means it interacts differently with the plant's chemical structure. For chemical lovers, DMSO forms a 1,4 addition, whereas alcohol forms a 1,2 addition. This distinction can influence how the plant's contents are removed and absorbed by the body.

I've used DMSO as a solvent to extract several plants, including cannabis, St. John's Wort, Arnica montana, calendula, horsetail, cayenne pepper, dandelion root, and many others. The outcomes have been outstanding. These DMSO extracts frequently have a greater transdermal (through the skin) effect than oil extracts. For further synergy, I prefer to mix DMSO and oil extracts, which appears to increase their efficiency even more.

This field of research—using DMSO as a solvent for herbal medicine—deserves far greater attention. It's mostly untapped, yet has enormous promise. However, unless you are well-versed in both plants and chemistry, it is usually better to leave the complex experiments to the professionals. After all, knowing how solvents interact with plant components and predicting the results is a science in itself.

Whether you're using colloidal silver or plant extracts with DMSO, the key is to understand how they operate and use them safely and efficiently. The possibilities are endless, and with proper use, they may be quite beneficial.

Using DMSO with Vitamin C: A Simple Guide.

When it comes to keeping our bodies in control, particularly in the prevention of cancer, DMSO paired with vitamin C provides a unique approach. Let us break things down in a way that is simple to grasp and use.

Our bodies are constantly on the hunt for intruders such as cancer cells. Fortunately, when everything works properly, such as our lymphatic system and overall health, our bodies can easily repair and replace damaged cells. Now here is where vitamin C and DMSO come into play.

Why combine DMSO with vitamin C? Vitamin C, commonly known as ascorbic acid, works similarly to glucose in human cells. Because our cells are always hungry for glucose (it serves as their fuel), they will readily absorb vitamin C. When you add DMSO to the mix, it improves vitamin C absorption, ensuring that it reaches the cells where it may be most effective.

If you feel like you're coming down with anything, such as a cold, a tiny dosage of vitamin C combined with DMSO may be precisely what your immune system needs. However, while taking bigger amounts, it is essential to select the appropriate type of vitamin C, especially if you are concerned about cancer prevention.

Choosing the Right Vitamin C Vitamin C comes in a variety of forms, some of which work better when mixed with DMSO. Buffered vitamin C, which is connected to minerals such as calcium or potassium, is gentler on your system and more effective at preventing sickness. Calcium ascorbate combined with a small amount of potassium ascorbate is an excellent choice for cancer prevention and overall wellness. These kinds of vitamin C are soft on the stomach and will not raise your salt levels, which is vital if you're trying to control your blood pressure.

How to Use DMSO with Vitamin C First, you must clean up your diet by eliminating processed sugar, white bread, and other items that might interfere with vitamin C absorption in your cells. You want to ensure that your cells are prepared to absorb all of that beneficial vitamin C rather than being distracted by sugars.

Here's an easy procedure to follow:

Vitamin C Dosage: Take 5 grams of buffered vitamin C twice day.

DMSO Dosage: Take 1 teaspoon of pure 99.995% DMSO combined with 5 ounces of distilled water or juice about 10 minutes before your second dosage of vitamin C. Begin with a ¼ teaspoon of DMSO and gradually increase to a full teaspoon over several days to allow your body to adjust.

Take DMSO on an empty stomach, either two hours after eating or two hours before the next meal. This will allow the DMSO to perform its job without hindrance.

A Few Important Tips:

Ease in: Increase your DMSO dosage gradually to minimize stomach discomfort. If you experience any pain, adhere to the lesser dose until your body adjusts to it.

Cycle the protocol: Use this regimen for two weeks at a time, about four times a year. This not only helps to prevent cancer, but it also offers your body a gentle cleanse and improves your immune system, allowing you to fight off colds and the flu.

DMSO and MSM: A Powerful Healing Combination

Let's discuss about MSM (methylsulfonylmethane), a naturally occurring substance that is extremely beneficial to your health. MSM may be found in plants, animals, and even common herbs like horsetail. In the lab, MSM is generated from DMSO, making the two an ideal fit when combined.

MSM is recognized for its anti-inflammatory effects, making it an ideal treatment for tendonitis, rheumatoid arthritis, and osteoarthritis. It benefits the skin, hair, nails, and even blood vessels because of its function in collagen formation. Additionally, unlike DMSO, MSM does not leave you smelling like garlic or oysters, which is always a bonus!

But why combine DMSO and MSM, especially if your body transforms some of the DMSO into MSM anyway? The answer is in their combined might. DMSO excels in penetrating tissues and transporting other compounds deeper into your cells. When used with MSM, it can help treat more serious illnesses such as Lyme disease, lupus, and cancer. There is continuing study into how these two can be combined in treatments, such DMSO Potentiation Therapy, which mixes DMSO with other compounds such as vitamin C and chlorine dioxide to enhance their effects.

How to Use DMSO with MSM

To minimize unpleasant detox effects, it is better to start with MSM gradually. Begin with 500 milligrams of MSM twice day, either in powder or pill form. Over the course of a few days, gradually increase the dosage until you're taking roughly half a teaspoon twice a day. If you're targeting a specific condition, you can increase to a full teaspoon twice a day. You may take MSM with or without meals; I've never had any trouble taking it on an empty stomach.

You can combine DMSO with MSM to have an even stronger impact. Begin with half a teaspoon of DMSO dissolved in 5 ounces of water or juice, then increase the MSM dose gradually. Personally, I love MSM in crystal form—they resemble huge bath salts. I just sprinkle the dry MSM crystals on my tongue and wash them down with some organic juice.

This combination is extremely powerful against parasites. DMSO helps to open up pathways for MSM to perform its work, making life difficult for unwelcome guests while also repairing your gut lining. Don't be shocked if you see benefits in your hair, nails, skin, and digestion within a week or two after beginning this treatment.

DMSO and Herbal Remedies: An Ideal Combination for Natural Healing

Dimethyl sulfoxide, or DMSO, has become a popular therapy for pain relief, inflammation reduction, and faster healing. However, when combined with natural medicines, it becomes much more effective. This combination combines the best of both worlds—

modern science and traditional wisdom—for a natural and effective approach to wellbeing.

Herbal Remedies: Nature's Medicine Cabinet

Herbal treatments have been used for centuries to help people recover and keep healthy via the power of plants. Herbs, whether in the form of a soothing cup of chamomile tea or a strong echinacea tincture, have several advantages. They can reduce inflammation, enhance the immune system, and even kill germs. These natural treatments have lasted the test of time because they are effective.

Why do DMSO and herbal remedies work so well together?

When you mix DMSO with herbal medicines, something wonderful happens. DMSO serves as a supercharger, allowing your body to absorb the healing compounds in herbs more efficiently. It's like giving those herbal remedies VIP access to where they're most needed.

Imagine you have painful muscles or hurting joints. Using a blend of DMSO and herbal extracts on your skin allows the healing properties to penetrate more deeply and quickly, offering fast relief. But it's not limited to just external use—when taken with herbal supplements, DMSO enhances their effectiveness, helping your body absorb more of their beneficial nutrients.

This combination is a natural powerhouse, allowing your body to better absorb the healing properties of herbs, whether you're fighting a cold, relaxing tight muscles, or simply wanting to stay healthy.

Common Herbal Remedies: Combined with DMSO.

DMSO, when paired with certain herbal medicines, can be a game changer for a variety of health problems. Let's look at some of the most successful combinations for naturally improving your mood.

Arnica: If you've ever had bruises, sprains, or muscular stiffness, you may be familiar with Arnica Montana. It is known for its anti-inflammatory and pain-relieving effects. Consider mixing it with DMSO as a topical cream or gel. The DMSO helps the arnica penetrate deeper into your skin, providing speedier relief from pain and swelling. This combination might help you recover faster after a strenuous workout or a fall.

Turmeric's active ingredient, curcumin, is well-known for its anti-inflammatory and antioxidant properties. Mixing turmeric extract with DMSO produces a strong remedy for joint discomfort, particularly for people suffering from arthritis. The DMSO guarantees that curcumin goes deep into your tissues, offering the comfort you seek.

Calendula, sometimes known as marigold or Calendula officinalis, is a skin-soothing plant. When combined with DMSO, it is an excellent treatment for small burns, wounds, and irritations. The DMSO allows the calendula to perform its magic directly on the afflicted region, speeding up healing and decreasing inflammation.

Ginger is well-known for its ability to soothe upset stomachs, but it also works wonderfully on tight muscles. Ginger, when mixed with DMSO in a cream or oil, can help relieve muscular pain and stiffness, making it an effective treatment for fibromyalgia and tension headaches. The warming feel of ginger, combined with the deep-penetrating action of DMSO, provides calming comfort exactly where it aches.

Safety Concerns and Precautions

While combining DMSO and herbal medicines might give a natural health boost, employ them carefully. Always consult a healthcare expert before beginning any new treatment, especially if you are taking medication or have allergies. To avoid skin irritation, DMSO should be appropriately diluted, and it is better to follow specified parameters for safe usage.

Acupuncture and DMSO: A Dynamic Duo.

Combining acupuncture with DMSO may not be the first thing that comes to mind, but the combination provides a unique technique to manage pain, decrease inflammation, and increase general well-being.

Understanding Acupuncture

Acupuncture, a crucial component of Traditional Chinese Medicine (TCM), is inserting small needles into certain places on the body to restore the flow of energy, or "qi." Acupuncture helps to balance the body's systems by treating certain spots, which relieves pain and promotes healing.

How DMSO Improves Acupuncture.

Acupuncture's benefits can be amplified when combined with DMSO. Applying DMSO to the skin before acupuncture helps minimize inflammation and irritation, making needle placement easier. Furthermore, DMSO's capacity to promote blood flow complements acupuncture's emphasis on energy channels, which may enhance the overall impact.

Following your acupuncture appointment, using DMSO topically can assist in extending the treatment's benefits. It promotes tissue healing and reduces post-treatment discomfort, offering long-term relief.

Potential Benefits and Considerations

Combining Acupuncture with DMSO for Pain and Healing

The combination of acupuncture with DMSO results in a powerful strategy for treating musculoskeletal pain, arthritis, sports injuries, and nerve diseases. This combo works by addressing two primary issues: energy imbalances and inflammation. Acupuncture restores the body's energy flow, whereas DMSO immediately decreases inflammation. Together, they provide a more comprehensive sort of comfort.

However, before beginning any therapy, you should exercise caution and check with a physician. When used appropriately, acupuncture and DMSO are both typically safe, although individual reactions may differ. A skilled practitioner should administer acupuncture, and while DMSO is helpful, it should be used with caution to avoid skin irritation or other negative effects. Always be aware of any underlying health issues or drugs that may interact with either therapy.

Ayurveda and DMSO: Integrating Ancient Wisdom with Modern Science

Ayurveda, India's time-honored medical tradition, and DMSO, a contemporary molecule known for its medicinal properties, may appear to be an unlikely combination. However, integrating the two provides a new approach to wellbeing. Let's look at how the old methods of Ayurveda may be enhanced by the qualities of DMSO, resulting in a unique marriage of tradition and science.

What is Ayurveda?

Ayurveda, which means "the science of life," focuses on establishing bodily equilibrium. It teaches that every one of us possesses a unique combination of three vital forces known as doshas: Vata (air and ether), Pitta (fire and water), and Kapha (earth and water). These doshas affect how we feel physically, cognitively, and emotionally. When the doshas are disrupted by stress, food, or other causes, the body becomes more susceptible to sickness. The purpose of Ayurveda is to restore balance via tailored therapies such as food changes, herbal medications, and lifestyle modifications.

Where Does DMSO Come In?

DMSO, well-known for its pain-relieving and anti-inflammatory properties, supports Ayurvedic therapy in a variety of ways. Here's how.

Enhancing Herbal Remedies: Ayurveda frequently uses herbal mixtures to treat a variety of diseases. When combined with these herbal oils, DMSO serves as a carrier, allowing the herbs to enter deeper into the skin or tissues. For example, combining Ayurvedic oils for joint pain with DMSO may assist in accelerating recovery by delivering therapeutic components directly to the location of suffering.

Boosting Detoxification: Ayurveda places a high value on detoxification to rid the body of toxic pollutants. DMSO supports this process by increasing circulation and decreasing inflammation, making it simpler for the liver to eliminate waste. When utilized intelligently in detox procedures, DMSO can boost the body's natural detox processes, resulting in greater overall health.

Practical Uses of Ayurveda with DMSO

Combining Herbal Oils and DMSO: If you currently use Ayurvedic oils to relieve pain or inflammation, adding DMSO can improve their effectiveness. Just be sure to start with a modest dose of DMSO and see how your skin reacts. The DMSO helps to push the herbal compounds deeper into the tissue, potentially resulting in faster alleviation.

Supporting Detox with DMSO: Adding DMSO to an Ayurvedic detox regimen will help your body clear toxins more effectively. Its capacity to promote circulation and decrease inflammation is ideally aligned with Ayurvedic detoxification aims. As usual, consult a medical practitioner to check that this combination is safe for you.

Important Considerations:

While combining DMSO with Ayurveda might be useful, it must be done under the supervision of a trained Ayurvedic practitioner and a DMSO-experienced healthcare professional. Both therapies have their own set of safety considerations, with DMSO, in particular requiring tiny dosages initially to watch for any adverse responses.

DMSO and Physical Therapy: A Powerful Combination for Healing

Thinking outside the box might help you deal with pain and inflammation. One intriguing way is to combine DMSO with physical therapy, resulting in a potent combination that accelerates healing and promotes general health.

What Physical Therapy Offers:

Physical therapy focuses on improving mobility, restoring function, and lowering pain using focused exercises, manual therapy, and other modalities. A physical therapist creates a unique strategy for each patient, concentrating on muscular strength, joint mobility, and flexibility. It's a hands-on approach to addressing the underlying causes of discomfort.

DMSO's ability to decrease inflammation makes it an excellent companion for physical therapy, resulting in improved pain relief. When combined, you get the best of both worlds: DMSO reduces swelling, while physical therapy strengthens the damaged region.

Faster repair: Ultrasound and electrical stimulation are common procedures used in physical therapy to improve tissue repair. Adding DMSO to the mix can improve this impact by promoting cellular regeneration, potentially shortening your recovery period.

Improved Range of Motion: If joint stiffness is limiting your mobility, DMSO can assist by boosting blood flow and decreasing inflammation. This makes physical therapy more effective in improving your flexibility and range of motion.

Quicker Recovery after Injury: Whether you're coping with a sports injury or recuperating from surgery, combining DMSO with physical therapy can help you recover quicker. DMSO's pain-relieving effects make it simpler to stick to rehab activities, which can result in faster development.

Holistic Care: By combining DMSO and physical therapy, you may address both the symptoms and the root causes of your pain. This holistic approach includes not only your physical health but also your emotional well-being.

How to Integrate DMSO with Physical Therapy

Topical Application: DMSO may be administered directly to the skin, and many physical therapists employ DMSO-based lotions or gels during sessions. Applying DMSO before exercise or manual treatment can assist the healing effects in penetrating deeper tissues.

Complementary Modalities: Physical therapy frequently employs instruments such as ultrasonography or electrical stimulation. DMSO can improve these therapies, allowing for greater outcomes in less time.

Home Care: Physical therapists frequently prescribe exercises that may be continued at home. By administering DMSO before completing your home workouts, you may be able to maximize the advantages and promote a speedier recovery.

Collaboration: To achieve the best results, your DMSO and physical therapy treatments should be carefully coordinated. This implies that your physical therapist and DMSO provider must collaborate to ensure that their treatments complement one another.

A New Frontier in Natural Healing

In preparation for this book, I researched every DMSO resource I could find, but none provided clear, easy-to-follow methods for creating DMSO mixes at home. That is why I am so thrilled to share this chapter with you. It contains unique DMSO recipes that you won't find anywhere else—at least not in the same format. These formulations combine DMSO with a variety of natural remedies, leveraging my extensive botanical knowledge, chemical expertise, and years of personal and professional experience making medications. The combinations you'll discover here aren't just modifications of existing concepts; they're created from scratch, combining the best of both traditional and modern methods of healing. I hope you will not only utilize these recipes with confidence but also remember this chapter as a useful resource. Feel free to mark it up, make notes, and pass it on through the generations. However, like with all changes to your health regimen, it's always a good idea to talk with a holistically educated healthcare professional before doing anything new. This book aspires to be more than simply a guide; it's meant to be a valued companion on your path to improved health. DIY Antifungal and Analgesic Solutions: Simple Recipes for Effective Relief If you're battling with troublesome fungal infections or persistent discomfort, homemade cures can be a game changer. Here's how to make some excellent antifungal drops and a potent analgesic mixture right in your kitchen. Antifungal drops are a simple solution for fungal issues. Ingredients: A 100 mL glass dropper bottle.1 mL of Lugol's Iodine or Povidone-Iodine44 mL of 99.995% pharmaceutical-grade DMSO.55 mL of distilled water. These antifungal drops are effective at treating toenail fungus, athlete's foot, jock itch, and even fungal diseases in dogs. They're an excellent go-to cure for those pesky fungal infections. Steps to

Make Antifungal Drops: Prepare your bottle: Begin with a clean 100-mL glass dropper bottle. Mix the ingredients: Add 1 mL of Lugol's iodine (or Povidone-iodine), 44 mL of DMSO, and 55 mL of distilled water to the container. Shake It Up: Screw on the cap and shake the bottle extensively to mix the contents. To maintain its effectiveness, store it at room temperature in a dark cabinet. How to use: For toenail fungus, Wash the affected area thoroughly with mild soap. Apply one to two drops twice a day, covering the nail and surrounding skin. Be patient; full recovery might take up to six months. For athlete's foot, soak your feet in a 50% apple cider vinegar solution for five minutes and then thoroughly dry them. Apply 1 to 2 drops between your toes and any sensitive skin regions twice a day. If feasible, clean your sporting shoes on a regular basis to prevent reinfection. Analgesic Formula: Natural Pain Relief. Ingredients: 50 mL glass dropper bottle. Mortar and pestle, or a zip-top bag with a rolling pin with 30 dried cloves.99.995% pharmaceutical-grade DMSO. This analgesic combination, which contains cloves and DMSO, is excellent for treating toothaches, muscular pain, and nerve pain. Cloves have long been recognized for their pain-relieving effects, and DMSO increases their potency. Steps to Create Your Analgesic Formula: Prepare the cloves: Lightly smash 30 dried cloves using a mortar and pestle or a zip-top bag and rolling pin. Combine Ingredients: Put the crushed cloves in a 50 mL glass dropper vial and fill with DMSO. Shake the bottle every single day for a week. After seven days, drain the cloves and return the liquid to the bottle. Keep it at room temperature in a dark area. To relieve tooth pain, apply 1 or 2 drops to the afflicted region 2-3 times per day, or as needed. If the discomfort persists, you may need to administer drops more regularly until relief is obtained. For muscle or nerve pain, combine 14 drops of the recipe and 6 drops of purified water or preservative-free aloe vera gel. Use this combination on the afflicted region up to four times per day. With black salve: To improve the absorption of black salve, combine 1 tablespoon of the analgesic mixture with 3 drops of eucalyptus and camphor essential oils, 2 drops of iodine, and 1 teaspoon of gum turpentine. Apply this combination to your skin before applying the black salve.

How to Make and Use DMSO Eye and Ear Drops

Eye Drops

Making your eye drops using DMSO is simple, but you have to ensure that everything is clean to keep your eyes safe and healthy. This is a step-by-step instruction for making your own DMSO eye drops.

Ingredients:

30 mL glass dropper bottle.

118 mL of distilled water.

Use ¼ teaspoon of non-iodized sea salt.

6.25 milliliters of 99.995% pharmaceutical-grade DMSO.

Instructions:

Sterilize Your Equipment:

Disassemble the dropper bottle.

Boil a saucepan of water, then carefully lower the bottle parts into it with tongs or a spoon.

Boil for 5 minutes, then remove and allow to air dry on a clean cloth or drying rack.

Reassemble the dry components using clean hands or gloves. Keep the lid on when making the solution to avoid contamination.

Prepare the solution.

Heat the distilled water in a kettle and dissolve the sea salt.

Using a syringe, add DMSO to the dropper bottle.

Pour 23.75 milliliters of saltwater solution into the bottle.

Replace the cap and shake the bottle. The interaction between DMSO and water causes the solution to warm up.

You have now prepared a 20% DMSO saline eye solution. For a 40% solution, just double the DMSO and adjust the saline concentration appropriately.

To use the eye drops properly, wash your hands with soap and water beforehand.

To avoid infection, do not contact your eyes or the dropper tip. If you accidentally contact it, thoroughly clean it with hot, soapy water before drying it with a clean towel or paper towel.

Label and date the bottle. Create a fresh batch every six months.

In a pinch, the 20% solution may be used as ear drops, but I recommend following my ear drop formula for the greatest results.

Learn how to produce ear drops with DMSO and colloidal silver.

Ingredients:

50 mL glass dropper bottle.

5 milliliters of 99.995% pharmaceutical-grade DMSO.

45 milliliters of 15 ppm colloidal silver.

Instructions:

Mix the ingredients.

Add the DMSO and colloidal silver to a clean dropper bottle.

Cap the bottle and gently shake it.

Before utilizing the combination, let it cool down from the first heat reaction.

For best results, apply 1-2 drops to each ear daily for a week.

When symptoms improve, continue taking the drops for a few more days to ensure the problem does not reoccur.

Label and date the bottle. Refresh the solution every six months.

These drops are intended to treat ear troubles by combining a 10% DMSO solution with colloidal silver. They are simple to produce and can give excellent relief when taken appropriately.

DMSO: Simple Solutions for Sinus Rinses, Wound Care, and Mouthwash.

When paired with other therapies, dimethyl sulfoxide (DMSO) can be a very effective tool in your health repertoire. Here's how to use DMSO effectively in sinus rinses, wound care, and mouthwash.

Sinus Rinse

What You Need:

Neti pot or nose spray bottle?

8 ounces of distilled water.

1/4 teaspoon neti salt or non-iodized sea salt

11 mL of 99.995% pharmaceutical-grade DMSO.

½ teaspoon 15 ppm of colloidal silver.

½ teaspoon of preservative-free aloe vera gel juice (optional).

How to Prepare:

Start with clean water: To avoid bacterial infection, rinse with lukewarm distilled water. If only tap water is available, boil it for three minutes and then cool until lukewarm.

Mix the solution. Stir the neti salt or non-iodized sea salt into the lukewarm water until thoroughly dissolved. Add the DMSO and mix carefully. Add the colloidal silver (with a plastic or wooden spoon, not a metal spoon).

Optional step: If the combination irritates, add ½ teaspoon of aloe vera gel juice to calm the nasal tissues.

Rinse: Apply the solution using a Neti pot or nasal spray bottle. Use this rinse only if your nasal passages are not raw or bleeding.

Wound Spray

What you need:

100 mL glass spray bottle.

50 mL of 99.995% pharmaceutical-grade DMSO.

50 milliliters of purified water or 15 parts per million colloidal silver

How to Prepare:

Mix the spray: Using a funnel, fill the spray container with DMSO and distilled water. If you want, use 50 mL of 15 ppm colloidal silver instead of water.

Storage and Use: Keep the spray in a cool, dry area. Use it on wounds after the bleeding has stopped. Avoid using it on surgical wounds containing sutures since it may dissolve them.

I recall my kid taking a bad crash while learning to ride her bike. She scraped her knee fairly badly. At first, I used our regular medicines, but the wound was taking too long to heal. I decided to test a 50% DMSO solution. To our astonishment, it did not hurt at all, and she felt instantly relieved. We used it three times every day, and the wound healed rapidly without leaving any scars.

Mouthwash

What you need:

3.5 mL of 99.995% pharmaceutical-grade DMSO.

3.5 mL of 3% food-grade hydrogen peroxide.

7 mL pure water or a combination of distilled water and preservative-free aloe vera gel juice

How to Prepare:

Mix your mouthwash: In a small bottle, combine DMSO, hydrogen peroxide, and distilled water (or a combination including aloe vera gel juice).

Use: Swish the mixture about your mouth for a few minutes before spitting it out. Use it twice a day, but do not swallow it.

Tip: Address the underlying cause of tooth problems, such as a poor diet or vitamin deficiency. Consider using remineralizing toothpaste or incorporating supplements like boron, magnesium, and vitamin K2 into your daily regimen.

DIY Scalp Care and Hair Growth Spray

If you're seeking for a simple but effective solution to improve scalp health and promote hair growth, this DIY spray might be your new best friend. I've had so many individuals tell me how much they enjoy this recipe for its ability to not only promote hair growth but also treat dandruff oil imbalances and even eliminate gray hairs. This is a simple recipe you can make at home.

What You Will Need:

A 100-milliliter glass spray bottle

50 milliliters of 99.995% pharmaceutical-grade DMSO.

20 milliliters of preservative-free aloe vera gel juice

30 milliliters of distilled water

6 drops of pure rosemary essential oil.

4 drops of pure peppermint essential oil.

How to Make It:

Begin by putting the DMSO into your spray bottle with a funnel to prevent spillage.

Combine the aloe Vera gel juice and distilled water.

Finally, add the rosemary and peppermint essential oils.

Give the bottle a brisk shake to blend everything together.

To use, spray the solution on clean, dry hair and scalp. To achieve the greatest results, start with a natural shampoo and conditioner. Apply enough sprays to cover not just the problem region but also some of the surrounding scalp. Allow the spray to soak completely. Remember to shake the bottle before each use thoroughly. For people suffering from long-term hair loss difficulties such as alopecia or male pattern baldness, consistency is essential—applying once or twice a day can make a difference over time. Just bear in mind that significant development may take many months, if not a year, so patience is key here.

Topical Vitamin and Mineral Blend

If you enjoy DIY skincare, this topical combination may be precisely what you need to help heal your skin or target particular problem areas. It's full of critical vitamins and minerals, all combined with the magic of DMSO to improve absorption and efficacy.

What you'll need:

A 50 mL glass dropper bottle.

1 milliliter of magnesium oil.

2 drops of Lugol's Iodine or Povidone-Iodine

Powder from 1/2 a vitamin C tablet

Powder from half a pill of a B-complex vitamin

40 milliliters of 99.995% pharmaceutical-grade DMSO.

10 milliliters of preservative-free aloe vera gel juice

How to Make It:

Using a funnel, pour the magnesium oil, iodine, and vitamin C and B-complex capsule powders into the dropper bottle.

Pour in the DMSO and aloe vera gel juices.

Shake the bottle well to ensure that everything is properly mixed.

Maintain your mix in a cold, dark area, and prepare a new batch every six months to keep it powerful. To use, apply 3 to 5 mL of the solution to any region of your body that needs additional healing care once or twice a day. Once you've mastered this basic combination, feel free to experiment by adding additional vitamins or minerals to meet your specific needs.

Crafting Your Own DMSO Creams and Gels at Home

Making your own DMSO creams and gels at home is a simple and cost-effective approach to benefit from the therapeutic properties of this versatile substance. With a few basic ingredients and a little ingenuity, you may create bespoke formulas that address your individual requirements right from the comfort of your own kitchen.

Choosing the Right Ingredients.

One of the advantages of producing your own DMSO products is that you can control what goes into them. Begin with a high-quality, pharmaceutical-grade DMSO solution, which you can get at health stores or online. You may then add different components based on your desired outcome.

Here are a few popular add-ins:

Aloe Vera Gel: Excellent for soothing and moisturizing the skin. Aloe vera can help relieve inflammation and speed up recovery.

Essential oils such as peppermint, lavender, and eucalyptus not only smell great, but they also provide pain relief and anti-inflammatory properties.

Arnica oil is an excellent remedy for bruises, sprains, and muscular pains, since it reduces pain and swelling.

Vitamin E Oil: Vitamin E, a potent antioxidant, protects your skin and promotes healing.

Menthol Crystals: Menthol is essential for relieving pain and inflammation because it provides a cooling sensation.

Easy DIY DMSO Creams and Gels

Ready to get started? Here are two basic recipes to try:

Basic DMSO Gel:

1/2 cup of aloe vera gel.

2 tablespoons of pharmaceutical-grade DMSO solution.

10 drops peppermint essential oil.

In a clean container, combine all of the ingredients and mix thoroughly. Keep your gel in a cold, dark place and use it when you need to relieve pain or inflammation.

Arnica-DMSO Cream:

1/4 cup Arnica oil

1/4 cup Shea butter

2 tablespoons of pharmaceutical-grade DMSO solution.

Ten drops of lavender essential oil.

Melt the arnica oil and Shea butter in a double boiler until smooth. Once it has cooled slightly, add the DMSO solution and lavender oil. Pour the cream into a clean container and keep it in a cold, dark place. Use this lotion to treat bruises and sprains or to calm tight muscles.

Make Your DMSO Solutions at Home

If you want to take charge of your health naturally, making your own DMSO solutions at home is an excellent place to begin. DMSO can help with pain, inflammation, and mild skin concerns. Plus, creating your solution is simple, inexpensive, and allows you to personalize it to your specific requirements.

Getting started with DMSO concentrations

Before you begin, let's discuss about DMSO concentrations. DMSO comes in a variety of strengths, often ranging from 70% to 99%. The solution becomes stronger as the concentration increases. But here's the catch: you shouldn't use it directly out of the bottle at full strength. It is critical to dilute DMSO correctly to avoid skin irritation or reactions. A decent rule of thumb is to begin with a lower concentration level and gradually increase as you get more comfortable.

Choosing the Right Ingredients.

To create your DMSO solution, you'll need high-quality, pharmaceutical-grade DMSO. You can get this at most health food stores or online. After that, the fun begins—you get to select extra elements that meet your demands.

Here are some typical elements to consider:

Distilled water: This is a necessity. Distilled water is clean and devoid of contaminants, making it an ideal basis for a DMSO solution.

Essential oils: Essential oils such as tea tree, lavender, and eucalyptus are excellent choices for additional benefits. They contribute their own set of therapeutic characteristics, such as lowering inflammation and combating germs.

Aloe Vera Gel: Known for its soothing and moisturizing properties, aloe vera gel can make your DMSO solution even gentler on the skin.

Witch Hazel: If you have oily or acne-prone skin, witch hazel is an excellent choice. It tones and cleanses the skin, maintaining its clarity and balance.

Simple Recipes to Get You Started

Let's look at a few simple dishes you may make at home:

Basic DMSO Solutions:

1 part pharmaceutical-grade DMSO.

Three parts distilled water.

Mix these in a clean container, and you're good to go. Keep your solution in a dark glass bottle to shield it from light, which might degrade the DMSO over time.

Antimicrobial DMSO Solution:

1 part pharmaceutical-grade DMSO.

One part distilled water

10 drops of tea tree essential oil.

Combine all of the ingredients in a jar to create a potent topical antibacterial. This mixture is ideal for treating small wounds, scratches, and even insect bites.

Safety First: What You Should Know

While producing your own DMSO solutions is typically safe, you should keep a few safety precautions in mind. Always use pharmaceutical-grade DMSO and ensure that all of your other components are of the highest quality. Before applying a new solution, perform a patch test on a small area of your skin to check there are no sensitivities or allergic responses.

Customizing Your DMSO Solutions.

Making your own DMSO solutions allows you to tailor them to your requirements, which is one of the most appealing aspects. Whether you want to cure, reduce inflammation, or simply pamper your skin, you may experiment with various components to see what works best for you.

Creating your own DMSO solutions at home is about more than simply saving money; it's also about taking control of your health in a natural and personalized way. So why not try it? You might be amazed at how effective and gratifying it is to make your own wellness treatments right in your home.

The Future of DMSO: Challenges and Opportunities.

DMSO, or dimethyl sulfoxide, has been around for decades, quietly establishing itself as a flexible and successful medicinal agent. However, like with any promising medicine, DMSO confronts both difficulties and potential as we move forward.

Overcoming Legal and Medical Barriers.

One of the biggest obstacles DMSO faces is the combination of legal and medical restrictions that have kept it from gaining wider acceptance. Despite its well-documented benefits, DMSO remains somewhat of an outsider in the medical world. The main reason for this is the lack of extensive clinical trials, which are typically required to secure broad approval in mainstream medicine.

That said, the landscape is gradually shifting. As more people seek out alternative and natural remedies, the interest in therapies like DMSO is growing. The path to overcoming these barriers lies in continued research and widespread education. By investing in studies that prove its effectiveness and safety, along with advocating for more openness within the medical field, we can help DMSO take its rightful place in today's healthcare system.

The Potential of DMSO in Modern Medicine

The potential for DMSO in modern medicine is immense. It has already showed promise in treating arthritis, inflammation, and several forms of cancer. What makes DMSO so appealing is its capacity to function as a carrier, improving the absorption and efficacy of other therapies. This offers up new opportunities for combining DMSO with other medications to develop potent, synergistic treatments.

Consider a future in which DMSO is commonly used in hospitals and clinics, not as a stand-alone therapy, but as part of a bigger therapeutic plan. For example, DMSO might be used with chemotherapy to help cancer medications penetrate cells more efficiently, thereby lowering the dosage and decreasing adverse effects. The possibilities are limitless, but attaining them will need a revolution in how the medical community perceives and uses this unique compound.

Advocacy and Education: How to Spread the Word

So, how can we get more people on board with DMSO? It begins with campaigning and education. As more individuals become aware of the benefits of DMSO, demand for its usage will increase. This is where personal tales and real-life experiences may make a significant difference. When individuals learn how DMSO has helped others, they are more inclined to consider it for themselves.

For those of us who believe in DMSO's potential, it is critical to spread the message. Every little bit helps, whether through social media, community discussions, or just sharing our experiences with friends and family. The more we discuss DMSO and its advantages, the more we can mainstream its usage and advocate for broader acceptance in the medical community.

In the end, the future of DMSO appears promising, but it is up to us to maintain the pace. By lobbying for greater research, educating others, and sharing our stories, we can help guarantee that DMSO realizes its full potential and becomes an important weapon in the fight for better health.

Conclusion

As we near the end of our journey through the wonders of DMSO, it becomes evident that this modest compound is much more than simply a tool for pain relief and inflammation reduction. DMSO draws on a long history of natural healing, combining age-old wisdom with current technology. Its flexibility is actually astounding, with advantages ranging from muscular relief to possible assistance for more serious health concerns. What distinguishes DMSO is not only its efficacy but also how it allows you to take control of your health in a natural and personalized way.

We've seen how DMSO may be used in a variety of ways, including as a simple homemade solution and as part of a more comprehensive health routine. It is an effective transporter, allowing other beneficial substances to enter deeper into tissues, making it an ideal complement to herbal therapies, essential oils, and other natural treatments. The potential of DMSO to improve absorption implies that you receive more out of your supplements and topical treatments, making them more effective with less effort.

However, the benefits of DMSO extend beyond physical wellness. There's something immensely fulfilling about taking a remedy that's been around for decades, one that's scientifically proven while being rooted in natural healing traditions. It serves as a reminder that the best answers are not always discovered in laboratories but rather in nature's medical cabinet.

When considering introducing DMSO into your health regimen, you should approach it with both curiosity and respect. While DMSO has several advantages, it is critical to use it responsibly, following rules and listening to your body. Begin carefully, try various applications, and pay close attention to how your body reacts. Everyone is different, and what works for one person may require some tweaking for another.

One of the most powerful characteristics of DMSO is that it restores your ability to heal yourself. You don't need sophisticated equipment or a chemistry degree to get the benefits of this remarkable substance. Whether you're making a basic remedy for a painful knee or looking into more complicated regimens for serious health issues, DMSO is a natural, effective, and accessible alternative.

In a world saturated with synthetic remedies with quick relief, DMSO stands out as a beacon of simplicity and efficacy. It's a tool that encourages us to slow down, reconnect with our bodies, and adopt a more natural approach to health. So, as you move forward, I encourage you to look into the possibilities that DMSO provides. Experiment with it, learn from it, and above all, listen to your body. The path to greater health is unique to each individual, and DMSO provides a dependable partner who is both adaptive and powerful.

Remember, perseverance and patience are essential components of any health journey. DMSO isn't a miracle cure, but it is a valuable friend in your search for health. By accepting this age-old understanding, you are not just treating symptoms but also nourishing your body in a natural, sustainable approach that is profoundly connected to nature's healing power. So, take the initial step, look into the possibilities, and believe in the process. Your body will thank you.